STUMBLE TO RISE

©**2019 Stumble to Rise** by Gina Whitlock Fletcher
Published by Rise Up Publishing

To obtain permission(s) to use material from this work, please e-mail your request to riseuppublishing@gmail.com.

ISBN: 978-1-7325015-0-8
e-ISBN: 978-1-7325015-1-5
Library of Congress Control Number: 2018967579

Editorial Services by Jerry Seidel and Kathleen Bambrick Meier
Cover Design by Shelby Weaver
Author Photo by Lauren Seidel Photography
Interior Design by Stephen Garrett

A portion of proceeds from book sales will be donated to Can Do Multiple Sclerosis.
To learn more about this organization visit:
https://www.cando-ms.org/

Printed in the United States of America

TABLE OF CONTENTS

Introduction

Chapter 1   The Adventure Begins   1

Chapter 2   Stumble, Recalculate, Adjust   19

Chapter 3   Moving On   35

Chapter 4   Losing the Pride   43

Chapter 5   Building a Toolbox   65

Chapter 6   Getting Behind the Wheel   75

Chapter 7   Recalculating   89

Chapter 8   Keeping It Simple   99

Chapter 9   Pre MS -- My Suit of Armor   115

Chapter 10   The Greatest Blessing   129

Chapter 11   Time to Rise   155

Conclusion   169

Acknowledgments   173

INTRODUCTION

Never let a stumble in the road be the end of your journey. ~
Unknown

Just as you are more than the set of circumstances
you've been dealt, I am more than Multiple Sclerosis, and I
refuse to be defined by it. For the first 10 years or so after
diagnosis, I attempted to obscure my disease from those around
me. The first impression of me was that of a healthy, vibrant
young woman. I was in a constant battle not only to hide my
condition but to eliminate it. MS didn't stand for that. As
symptoms have progressed, my MS is likely to be the first thing
one sees upon meeting me. When I'm using a mobility device it's
impossible to encounter me without noticing my condition first.

I recently viewed a documentary about disability in
this country. When I saw MS on the list of possible disabling
conditions, I was, to my husband's surprise, shocked. I hadn't
before considered myself as a person with a disability. Like my
fellow MS warriors, I'm a master at navigating my world with
an overwhelming set of challenges while most importantly,
maintaining a happy and hopeful outlook. If anything, that
proves I'm skillfully-ABLED which is the polar opposite of
DISabled. I've discovered that there isn't just one way to survive
and thrive. When the most obvious route becomes impassible,

there is another one ready to be traveled. While accepting some support along the way, it becomes our job to find that alternate path.

With MS, I've been forced to let go of old assumptions about my future. I've mourned those losses and look back at that old life with fondness -- the same way that anyone recounts now cobwebbed memories of another time. Rather than getting stuck in the loss of what was, I look ahead to continually rising and becoming the best possible version of a new me.

In the following pages, I share how I've struggled, taken control, and maintained a mostly joyful perspective in spite of those daily challenges. Even though I get frustrated by the changes happening in my body, I've taken powerful, transformative steps to regain a sense of control. After 23 years with MS, I realize that I am not fighting to make my disease disappear, but instead, I battle to make myself stronger than my disease.

If you are struggling to overcome what may be devastating realities in your own life, whether it's MS or something else, I hope to inspire you to keep moving forward. Through my greatest teacher, disguised as struggle, I've reinvented myself and have become a warrior. I hope my story inspires you to RISE above your own stumbles in the road.

Challenges are gifts that force us to search for a new center of gravity. Don't fight them. Just find a new way to stand.

~ Oprah Winfrey

*For my two guys who
bring me love, joy, and laughter every day.*

STUMBLE TO **RISE**

My Life Surviving and Thriving With MS

by Gina Whitlock Fletcher

CHAPTER ONE

The Adventure Begins

A strong woman has faith that she is strong enough for the journey...But a woman of strength has faith that it is in the journey that she will become strong.

~ Unknown

At 49 years old, I own three walkers, two canes, one wheelchair, and a mobility scooter. I never imagined any one of these devices being part of my daily life. However, it's human nature to take our abilities for granted until they are compromised or gone completely. I certainly did.

With my long legs, I used to maneuver quickly and with purpose. I never considered slowing down or conserving my energy. I strolled the mall, wore high heels, worked out, ran errands, and definitely never stressed about quickly finding a restroom. I could accomplish all of that and prepare a big dinner or be ready for an evening event with ease. I was unstoppable.

Fast forward to my current situation. Even with mobility aids, I walk like a drunk: zigzagging, stumbling constantly and falling once or twice daily. I must concentrate on every single step. When I am distracted and move too quickly, my feet don't necessarily continue in the intended direction. I'm likely to end up crashing to the ground or into a wall. As I no longer seem to have a graceful bone left in my body, I've sustained many injuries, with some requiring medical attention. Like a bare-legged toddler who's been climbing on the jungle gym, I'm usually peppered with black and blue bumps and bruises or worse. For example, at my recent 30 year high school reunion I appeared with one stylish boot that complimented a sexy outfit paired with a protective orthopedic boot to cushion my broken toes...the painful outcome of an awkward mishap the day before. Such things happen so regularly now that I can't even recall how they occur. It wasn't always this way.

This all began for me at the age of 27. I was happily married to my best friend and soulmate, engrossed in the beginning of a new career and feeling completely vibrant and healthy. I'd never before experienced any illness outside of the occasional cold or flu, so when a strange numbness in my right hand and forearm appeared one September morning, I quickly dismissed it. I must have slept in a strange position. We were, after all, out of town for a Labor Day weekend visit with my in-laws and sleeping on an uncomfortable sleeper sofa -- you know, the kind with a metal bar that runs across your back. My amateur diagnosis for this bizarre sensation was that the bar might have caused a nerve ending to twist. I was certain that the odd feeling would subside after a few days.

During this time of my life, I spoke daily to my mom and kept her in the loop about our comings and goings. My family was always very loving and tightly connected. As my siblings and I became adults, we all communicated through my mother who kept us informed about everyone else's activities. I heard about the happenings in my sisters' lives through Mom, and likewise, she would share my adventures with them. She was definitely the connective tissue binding us together from day to day.

In one such conversation with her around that time, I explained what was happening with my hand. She asked a few questions and then suggested I make an appointment with a neurologist as soon as we returned home. That seemed rather extreme, but since she had always been a worry wart, I took her loving advice to be the overreaction of a concerned mother.

After a few days had passed, the numbness and tingling did not subside but intensified. It was not only frustrating but annoying. When a client handed me money that included loose change, I heard the coins hit the wood floor but didn't realize they had fallen out of my hand until I saw them by my feet.

As I'm right-handed, nearly every simple task took on an extra level of effort: writing a note, brushing my teeth, grabbing a jar of pickles from the refrigerator. It was like that feeling when your electricity goes out yet you inadvertently try flipping the lightswitch on and off when you enter the room. A numb hand is the same. We take it for granted when it's completely operational, but when it's not, it's nearly impossible to remember that it's out of commission.

My sister called me to say our mother was worried and upset because she was afraid I might have multiple sclerosis. MS? Are you kidding me? How could she possibly jump to that conclusion based on one numb hand? Other than that, I felt fine.

My husband and I often joked that my mom had a touch of "Debbie Downer"- ism. We could be laughing and enjoying a funny moment when Mom, with impeccable timing, might interject the news of a fatal car accident in another town or an acquaintancès' sister's cousin who was admitted to the hospital yesterday.

However, after the call with my sister, I was slightly concerned. My mom was a walking medical encyclopedia. Throughout my life, she had a knack for correctly diagnosing the medical conditions of others. Whether it be immediate family, friends, her employees, or church members, everyone knew they could explain their symptoms to Mom, and she could often correctly diagnose them before any doc ever had the chance. Moreover, she would even give someone tips to better manage the symptoms temporarily until they got medical attention.

Her hunches were almost always accurate. However, when she wanted clarification, she referred to one of the many medical books she kept handy for easy reference. Albeit quite amateur, I think she thoroughly enjoyed this foray into the medical field and probably more so than if she had been an actual MD.

After learning of my mom's concern, I quickly decided to see a neurologist as soon as possible to pacify her and relieve her worries as well as mine. I desperately scanned the Yellow Pages with a mission to find a neurologist who could see me immediately.

Scheduling appointments with a specialist usually requires a wait of up to several months. At the time, I didn't know this. The only other specialist I'd ever seen was an oral surgeon when I had my wisdom teeth extracted. So I simply opened the phone book and found the lengthy list of neurologists whom I assumed would be readily available to see me. Beginning with the A's, I dialed each one -- no appointments available. So I moved on to the B's. When I make up my mind to accomplish something, I can be annoyingly tenacious until I've successfully completed the task. Just ask my husband. I was determined to call every single neurologist listed under every letter of the alphabet until I got an appointment. As luck would have it though, toward the end of the letter B's, I found a neurologist with a last-minute cancellation who could see me the very next day. Ignorance is often bliss, and sometimes, very lucky.

Despite my telling them it was no big deal, my parents made the drive from 90 miles away to be by my side for the appointment. They wanted to be with their baby girl, and while that was really sweet, it certainly made the situation even more intense.

My first-ever neurological exam was a comical experience. As Dr. B conducted it, I was mildly amused by the need to intently focus on his fingers while he asked how many he was holding up. Come on! Did he really think that counting would be difficult for me? I'm a college graduate. I can count; I just had some numbness. Then he used little metal tools, some of which vibrated, to bang on my limbs while asking me if I could feel them. I could feel everywhere he tapped and vibrated except my hand and forearm! Then he asked me to walk down the hallway as he watched and took notes. Not a problem. I assumed I had passed this last little test with flying colors too, and the doctor was still searching for answers. An MRI was scheduled for the next day.

I didn't have time for any of this! I was busy. I had appointments and phone calls to make. I was glad to see things were happening quickly so we could get this process over with, but I wasn't prepared for any of it, especially the MRI. I'll never understand why no one explained to me what to expect. While many adults are probably familiar with the procedure, I was completely clueless. I presumed that an MRI was similar to an x-ray. Boy, was I wrong.

First I had to get undressed and wear a paper towel robe. Then I was placed inside a long tube with my head bound within a tight cage. Meanwhile, I was instructed to lie perfectly still in this position for nearly two hours! This was all more than I could handle. The cacophony of noises that ensued was enough to bring me to tears. It sounded like deafening nuclear alert-warning signals combined with 25 jackhammers busting concrete two inches from my eardrums. Even though I was wearing headphones, the echoing racket was thunderous.

After a few torturous minutes in the tube, tears started rolling down the side of my face and pooled by my ears in little puddles. I couldn't move to wipe them, so I laid there feeling completely overwhelmed, helpless, soggy and frightened about what was happening to me. It was then I knew something was about to change, but I had no idea what was in store.

I can't imagine the hot mess that greeted the tech when he pushed the button on the little conveyor belt that rolled me out of the tube. When he removed the cage and saw my wet, mascara-stained face, he asked if I was okay.

Was I okay?! I had no idea! I hadn't been to a doctor in years, and now I was suddenly immersed in a slew of crazy tests, medical buildings, brain specialists, and co-pays with absolutely no understanding of what was happening to me.

Anyone who has anxiously awaited the outcome of a diagnosis knows that your imagination starts running rampant with doom and gloom life-altering possibilities. Maybe a pinched nerve was to blame, and I would undergo surgery followed by a long course of physical therapy. Perhaps I had brain cancer and would be given a life expectancy of six months or less; maybe even worse, a hidden brain aneurysm that could instantly burst and leave me dead within seconds. Or maybe it was nothing at all and would resolve itself like hiccups always do. Oddly, I remembered reading in a *Guiness World Records* book about an unfortunate fellow from Iowa who had suffered with hiccups for 68 years. Thankfully, for most of us, they vanish within an hour. Perhaps my numbness would, too, but I wanted information and didn't expect this process to take so long.

The day after the MRI, I was already calling Dr. B's office for results. In my world, when someone left me a message, I would call back within a few hours. I soon learned the medical field operated by a different set of rules. I left voicemail messages and begged for an earlier appointment with receptionists, office staff and medical assistants to no avail. The doctor, they informed me, would not tell me anything until my follow-up visit which was scheduled for three-and-a-half weeks later. No way could I wait three-and-a-half weeks to find out what the doctor already knew. I continued to call and plead, but they had no openings. I kept my mind occupied and was actually productive as I worked to pass the time between calls. With the predicted cadence of a soldier, I dialed that neurologist's office every two hours as I was determined to get in front of Dr. B ASAP. Even though I was persistent, I was respectful and kind. This was a technique I had perfected as the youngest sibling who was skilled at convincing others to succumb to my wishes. I had learned early on that you do, in fact, attract more flies with honey. So as irritating as my phone calls were becoming, I was laying it on thick with how much I appreciated each member of that office staff for their assistance. When they answered, I knew their names and would cheerfully say, "Hi Sue, it's me again!"

Soon they were pressuring the doctor to squeeze me in for a quick visit. His kind staff went to bat for me, leaving him notes and mentioning my name over and over. After a couple days of this routine, the phone rang on a rainy Thursday afternoon, and when I answered I certainly didn't expect to hear Dr. B's voice. I'm sure he'd grown tired of my name. There was no greeting and no chance to utter a word. He firmly stated his name and then bluntly jumped right to the point of the call.

"I have the results of your MRI, and it appears that you have multiple sclerosis." I remember those words echoing in my mind and then hearing an unexpected lingering silence from his end. I managed to weakly respond with one word: "Really?" That was the best response I could muster to a potentially life-changing diagnosis? He then continued by confirming that I would get more information at my scheduled appointment. He didn't ask if I had any further questions. He didn't indicate any details about what was on my MRI. He said he would see me in three weeks and curtly disconnected. That was it. One of the most monumental conversations I'd ever had was over in less than 60 seconds.

On the verge of tears, I immediately called Scott and shared the news with him. His knowledge of MS was even less than mine, but he reassured me that whatever happened he would be there with me every step of the way, and we would figure it out together.

The wedding vows we'd taken just four short years earlier seemed strikingly fitting on that day. It crossed my mind that if I became completely dependent on Scott, he might choose to rethink that "in sickness and in health" commitment. He had said "I do" to a healthy, independent young woman. He hadn't bargained for a defective disease-stricken wife this quickly. If he had purchased a new car that shortly thereafter turned out to be a lemon, he would at least have a bumper to bumper warranty that might include a total replacement. With me, there were no exchanges or returns, and I hoped he didn't grow to feel "stuck" in a caregiver role.

Multiple sclerosis was exactly what my mother had predicted, so I called her next and confirmed that her suspicion had been correct. She got my dad on the phone, and I could hear and feel their combined disappointment and unconditional love enveloping me over the phone line. Later, through my own research and at the follow-up appointment, it was confirmed that what my medically-savvy mother had sensed all along was true. I perfectly fit the textbook profile of this disease. I was a 27-year-old white female who had randomly scattered lesions covering the brain and spinal cord. The clarity of my situation had made for a slam-dunk diagnosis.

The next day, my natural hopefulness and confidence was shaken, so I immersed myself into all the MS research I could find. Of course, this was long before Google or WebMD existed which meant multiple trips to the bookstore and the library. Over the next 48 hours, I set up a mini research lab in the kitchen of our small apartment. I learned about a disease of the central nervous system that has no defined cause or cure and is unpredictable and unique to each individual based on the location of his or her specific lesions.

In a healthy human body, messages directing a desired action to your hands, legs, or bladder, for example, travel quickly and uninterrupted from your brain or spinal cord. In

11

someone with MS, the messages are interrupted on their path because the patient's body chooses to attack a coating on the nerves called myelin. Why this happens no one seems to know. MS isn't contagious or typically considered to be hereditary although it does have some repetitive family tendencies. To add to the confusion, I came to learn that doctors often had differing opinions on the best steps to take after diagnosis. The literature was full of random and fuzzy information, with one source often completely contradicting another. As I continued my reading, I discovered some people with the disease remained unaffected for the rest of their lives while others deteriorated quickly with complications leading to early death. Any number of body systems could be compromised or possibly none at all.

The more I learned, the more confused and concerned I became. I was coming to the conclusion that this was a completely wacky and unpredictable disease. I certainly wasn't finding the clarity that I craved to instill confidence about my future.

By the next day, which was a sunny and unseasonably crisp mid-September Sunday, Scott and I were mentally and emotionally drained. A break from everything MS-related was needed -- something totally carefree and outside of our typical routine.

We headed to a theme park we hadn't visited in years. Here, perhaps, would be some youthful fun and distraction.

When we arrived and parked in the massive lot, we both noticed an inordinate number of park visitors in wheelchairs or using other mobility devices. This seemed to be either a cruel joke or my mind was playing tricks on me.

I remembered learning in a college psychology class about the Baader-Meinhof phenomenon. It's a frequency illusion that occurs when you learn about something obscure and then you start seeing it everywhere you look. For example, if you start thinking about yellow cars after reading this, I guarantee you'll see yellow cars continually when you hit the road.

However, that theory was quickly squashed. As we approached the gate, we saw a banner above the entry turnstiles that read: "Handicap Awareness Day." The irony of that coincidence actually made us laugh which felt twistedly therapeutic after our previous 48 hours. I suppose that was a precursor to the humor that would be required later to navigate through all the MS muck in my future.

That day's attempt at diversion worked. Not only did I relish the light-hearted, much-needed fun, but the day proved that life was forging ahead for those around me. When we suffer a great blow or loss, we might forget that everyone else is still moving along in their ordinary routines as if nothing has happened at all.

With maturity, however, comes the realization that

everybody else is also dealing with their own conflict or uncertainty about something. Looking back, I'm positive that the other park visitors using mobility aids to transport themselves around that sprawling place were, like me, trying to divert their attention, albeit for only a few hours, from their daily reality. We don't always consider that as we are absorbed in our own situations.

Now that I'd survived the first few days post-diagnosis, I engrossed myself in routine and didn't mention what had just transpired to anyone outside of my inner circle. If someone asked what I'd been doing all weekend, I was quick to say, "Not much, how about you?"

Once the three weeks passed, my husband and my parents attended the follow-up office appointment armed with my mom's lengthy list of detailed questions prepared for this elusive doctor with his subpar bedside manner. She was the person you wanted by your side digging for answers at an important medical appointment.

Dr. B certainly offered no comfort and didn't seem to realize that even though this situation was a daily occurrence for him, it was a once-in-a-lifetime blow for me. I remember glancing from Scott's and my dad's concerned faces to watching Dr. B's sullen face as he spoke, but I don't remember much that he said. His style was very technical, cold and compassionless, and he didn't seem to be accustomed to someone like my mother with her knowledgeable and very pointed questions.

My MRI films were lit up on a white box, and he casually pointed out all the patches that he referred to as plaques. I supposed that he had seen similar pictures many times before, but it seemed very surreal to me. It was impossible to comprehend that I was sitting in this strange office surrounded by people I loved while viewing the many flaws inside my brain and torso. It felt like I was suddenly thrust into the starring role of the only "medical" show I had ever watched, *General Hospital.* (I was never an *ER* or *Grey's Anatomy* fan.) "Would Gina survive this horrifying diagnosis? Would her handsome husband, Scott, stay with her or leave for a healthier woman? If he stays, will they become the 90's version of Luke and a handicapped Laura? Stay tuned to find out…"

I didn't hear many answers that made much sense, so at a certain point, I tuned out and stared at the industrial black and white clock on the wall. It reminded me of the ones in my grammar school classrooms. I watched the second hand as it barely crept along just like in 4th grade when it was almost time for lunch, and I thought the bell would never ring.

I snapped back into reality when Dr. B attempted to answer my mom's question about the likely trajectory of my disease. He didn't know. I may have more attacks of other body parts but when and if were big unknowns. He certainly gave me no expectations about the things that mattered for my future. He flippantly explained that it was a "wait and see" kind of disease. He offered little information, but my determined mother got him to open up about new drugs, needles, injections and side effects. We left the highly-anticipated appointment without much more detail than I'd already gained from reading a pamphlet in the office waiting room.

I had no idea what this unfamiliar disease entailed, and I was more confused after the appointment. My husband and I had only been married for a few years, and in spite of my normally confident outlook, we both had questions about our future. Could I continue my current career path? Would we be able to have children? The problem with questions about MS is that there are no answers, so while I am someone who craves clarity and control, this disease offers neither.

The image that I couldn't seem to shake was that of a poor soul confined to a wheelchair. However, I felt strong and invincible, so once I gained some distance from the depressing neurologist whom I vowed to never lay eyes on again. I believed I would somehow be the exception to such a miserable fate. I couldn't imagine it would ever be me in that wheelchair. Instead, I would learn everything about this condition, get a handle on controlling it, and would be just fine.

After that day I knew I couldn't continue to consume myself with this diagnosis. Though I now supposedly had a chronic disease of the central nervous system, I felt fine. The numbness and tingling was starting to fade a bit, so physically,

I felt no different than before the diagnosis. I was no MS victim! I was back to my strong, invincible, goal-setting self. Eventually, I got a second opinion, and the new neurologist explained that while MS was most likely correct, there was a possibility I had a strange MS step cousin. He mentioned terms like "transverse myelitis" and "clinically isolated syndrome" so until a second exacerbation appeared, I may or may not have MS or any of these oddly related conditions. I ran with the theory of "may not" and held tightly to the notion they had this whole thing all wrong with me.

This new doctor suggested I start on one of three new injectable drugs in an effort to prevent further progression if it was MS. However, no one was certain these drugs would actually work! In those days, the three new MS drugs didn't yet have years of clinical data behind them showing positive results. As I read the possible negative side effects -- fever, chills, body aches and pains, depression, and headaches -- my decision was clear. It was actually a no-brainer for me. I would completely skip the needles and focus on the one thing which all the doctors agreed upon: the best way to counteract any of this was maintaining an active lifestyle. With that information, I decided to fight and to take control of the situation. I would stay busy and focus on my new business. And, of course, I implemented a daily exercise program, joined a gym, and planned to prove both doctors wrong.

Like a child who plays baseball in the backyard and

imagines a stadium full of cheering fans, I envisioned I would someday be the wheelchair-free poster child of an action plan to completely annihilate MS through daily exercise. Maybe I would write a book and hit the talk show circuit forcing Dr. B to publicly apologize for his lack of knowledge.

Even though I was shaken, I was determined to prevail. I just knew I was going to be okay. I thank my father for instilling in me the calming belief that things will work out. He was the master of optimism and didn't waste a minute worrying. Thankfully, I inherited his perspective.

My mother on the other hand was highly skilled at sweeping things under the rug and ignoring their existence. For as long as I can remember, when we spoke about our own possible difficulties, she was adept at saying, "Let's not talk about that" and quickly changed the subject to something more pleasant. She didn't deny reality, but she certainly didn't want to welcome trouble before it arrived. Her philosophy was, "We'll cross that bridge when we get there." Like a good daughter, I suppose I combined their coping mechanisms and chose to move forward accordingly. Despite a future that now offered a new uncharted level of uncertainty and inherent difficulties, I knew in my heart that I would come out on top of this damning diagnosis. Though not offered any guarantees, somehow I was certain that I would RISE above MS!

CHAPTER TWO

Stumble, Recalculate, Adjust

We delight in the beauty of the butterfly, but rarely admit the
changes it has gone through to
achieve that beauty. ~ Maya Angelou

From the first breath we take to our last, our lifelong journeys are marked by a series of radical transformations. For the first year or so of a human life, babies aren't built to be mobile. As each child learns to walk, they must first endure repeated painful falls. It's the ultimate stumble-to-rise scenario.

It must be frustrating to watch others traipsing around easily while you're stuck crawling on the floor. But babies don't let discouragement stop them. They bend their crooked legs, attempt to pull themselves up, and put one tiny foot in front of the other until BOOM -- they come crashing down on their soft diapers yet again.

Eventually, after multiple unsuccessful attempts and sustaining a few bumps and bruises, nearly every one of us triumphantly figures it out. Some take a tad longer to conquer the skill, but I've never heard of one able-bodied little person who threw in the towel and accepted crawling as their primary mode of ambulation. They adjust and re-attempt until they're darting in all directions faster than their parents can follow.

Conversely, I've now witnessed the complete opposite scenario with my once strong and physically fit father. Because of Alzheimer's disease at the end of his life, he couldn't even transport himself from the bed to the toilet without the aid of a Hoyer lift or two strong helpers. The litany of radical changes that any one of us must endure over a lifetime could be the tumultuous plots of many engrossing novels or blockbuster movies. Change is undeniable. Other than death, it's the only guarantee we have. How we respond to it, however, may determine our happiness quotient.

For my mother's entire life, she had a terribly arduous time dealing with change. When it was finally time to help my mom clear out my childhood belongings, Mom froze in her avoidance of the ugly process and what it likely represented. She knew she would eventually have to leave the big family house that was so full of memories. Even though I was now an adult, she couldn't seem to rid her house of any shred of my past. For the nearly 30 years after leaving home, my bedroom remained a shrine to my youth. Every music box, trophy, stuffed animal and poster was in place, just as I'd left them. In fact, my husband, whose mother had excitedly emptied her home of his childhood leftovers shortly after he moved out, reminded me how bizarre it was that a 40-something married couple would still spend the night in the "Gina Museum" on family visits.

This scenario brings to mind a recent *Saturday Night Live* skit poking fun at what happens when young women bring their boyfriends home for the holidays. Covertly mashing with their beau under the watchful eyes of their teddy bears certainly made me giggle.

As I purged my old memories into piles of keep, donate and trash, Mom looked on as I sorted, and I encouraged her with these words, "Bless it and release it, Mom." However, it was as if she couldn't bear to let even the smallest memory go. Her instinct was to fight change, avoiding it even when it could bring improvement. For her, there was peace in constancy.

To spare her from enduring even more of this painful process, I eventually loaded everything into boxes and completed the sorting at home. Near the end of her life, the changes brought on by the progression of my dad's condition combined with her own declining health were massive and too hard for almost anyone to handle, but especially for her. Eventually, depression and worry plagued her constantly. I visited her often during that time and deemed my visits as joy-spreading missions. Often accompanied by my husband and young son, we brought games to play, sang songs, and had jokes on the ready with the goal of making her smile and celebrating when we got a laugh! Even during somber times, humor was always part of our survival.

In my own life, the transitions and ensuing adjustments have been plentiful. Just ten years ago both my parents were alive, healthy and active. I lived in a different house with a three-year-old son at my heels. I could walk confidently and maneuver with ease, and I was busily focused and achieving goals in a direct sales career. Now, every one of those realities has shifted.

As a young adult starting out after college graduation, I certainly didn't imagine that my experiences up to then were an invaluable dress rehearsal for the disjointed circumstances that would eventually transpire. My then boyfriend, Scott, and I were college graduates proudly armed with our diplomas and contributing to the unemployment rate of the post-cold war recession. In addition to our own wedding planning and my dream-come-true summer stint as the vocalist for The Ronnie Scott Orchestra, a 12-piece swing band, we were mailing resumes and filling out applications daily. Simply securing an interview was incredibly difficult at that time. As much as I loved my stage time with the group, I knew it wasn't stable or practical for a soon-to-be-married woman to travel around the state in a van with a bunch of musicians for weekend gigs. I needed a legitimate "grown-up" career.

When neither of us could find employment, our naive hopes of early financial success had to be seriously readjusted. My kind parents eventually "found" jobs for us at one of their businesses in a small central Illinois town. They provided us a start when we didn't have many options.

Scott eventually landed a job in Chicago, and we traded the small town for the big city -- and the opportunity to finally get started as an independent couple. Shortly thereafter, I was hired as a headhunter for a staffing agency. I invested in suits and heels and worked in a high rise office building located in a bustling area. Working alongside a team of diverse and entertaining women who matched companies with applicants, gave me an in-depth introduction into the world of sales and cold calling. I spent several sedentary hours a day pounding the phones to land possible candidates and client companies. For lunch, a few of us would swap out our heels for sneakers and get moving. In those carefree pre-MS days, I thought nothing of a few vigorous treks up and down the 16 flights of stairs for a much needed break from the phones. (Never mind that we erased much of our 'gains' by trotting over to nearby restaurants to eat big unhealthy lunches and bring back sugary desserts to our desks.)

After a few years of hustling in that challenging draw-versus-commission pay structure, I was recruited by a client company. It was a business which had used our services to hire both temporary and permanent employees. Now working on the opposite side of the desk in human resources for the world headquarters of a manufacturing facility, I interviewed, selected and hired factory workers, accountants and engineers. I also directed employee orientations and dealt with daily workplace conflicts. I became good at it, but after controlling my own income in the staffing world, it was incredibly boring to receive the same predictable paycheck every two weeks. Though I knew it was merely a stepping stone to something with more individuality and potential, I still missed the thrill of being in control of my income. I was open to a career shift but had no idea where I would land.

Around that time, I was invited to a PartyLite get together by a former staffing company friend named Stephanie. This was the kind of home gathering where friends come together with a glass of wine, some appetizers and scrumptious desserts while socializing and shopping for scented candles and decor. I reluctantly showed up on a rainy, cold weeknight after Steph called at the last minute and begged me to attend. As she knew I was powerfully motivated by sugar, she lured me in with the promise of a decadent and fudgy dessert I could not resist.

Once there, I was intrigued by what the party rep had to say. She was self-employed, setting her own schedule and making more money than I was at a full-time job. I'd been raised in a very entrepreneurial home, so the freedom, flexibility and potential offered by this type of sales organization appealed to me.

Best of all, there was an escape hatch. I could give it a shot and if it didn't proliferate, I'd just keep my day job. It was a win-win situation. They offered a no cost option to get started, so no matter what happened, I would make some new friends, earn quick cash and end up with lots of great smelling candles.

I was off to a valiant start. I attended all available trainings, and within six months, I had built a team and earned a free cruise. I was too inexperienced to know these types of businesses often have a high failure rate. I simply did what I was told and saw big results.

An often forgotten benefit of youth is that we blindly forge ahead without allowing the fear of failure to stand in our way. Years later I heard it described as, "Ignorance on fire is better than knowledge on ice." I definitely proved that statement to be true.

As a result of my newfound success, the corporate grind was quickly losing its early appeal. This new avenue to becoming my own boss had me hooked. It offered high income growth and the ability to coach and inspire others to achieve their own goals just like I was doing. I was not only intrigued, but challenged by both. The free tropical vacations and countless rewards along the way were icing on the cake.

When my husband got a job offer in the St Louis area, we happily accepted the option to relocate six hours south. It was the excuse I'd been hoping for to leave the corporate grind and focus on my new candle gig. Making the move in March of 1995, we left Chicago and its cool spring morning air only to pull into St.Louis and its near tropical temps that afternoon. With temperatures close to 80 degrees, I wondered if I'd somehow been transported to the deep south. We rented a small apartment and enjoyed the adventure of starting over together in another new area.

The out-of-state move also meant leaving my newly-created team in Chicago. I'd built a small group of sellers there and enjoyed a bustling sales calendar, but with a move to a new state, everything came to a screeching halt. I only knew one person in St. Louis. Though my longtime best friend, Andrea, was nearby, my dream of making my mark on the direct sales world looked rather bleak. I was barely contributing to our household income with my fledgling business, and I began to question my objective. I was personifying the idea of "failing forward" on a daily basis. Doors were closed in my face at nearly every turn. Goals were set but frustratingly not reached. I heard the word "No" so many times that I became numb to it. I found that once I heard 10 No's, I would then, invariably, get a yes. The inconsistent pace of one step forward, two steps back continued. So I began tracking my rejections on lists, usually welcoming the negative responses with a smile. I didn't know it then, but I'm certain that persevering through that disheartened time in a new area set me up with the resiliency required for later challenges.

After a few months of discouragement, I took a part-time job in my old staffing field and despised it. My new coworkers were wonderful, but my boss, Mr. S, was a revolting caricature of an old-school chauvinist with alcoholic and narcissistic tendencies who provided additional inspiration to build my business and get out of there quickly.

That job represented my thus far failed attempt to make my own venture thrive. It didn't help matters that I was exactly like my dad. I didn't want a boss, and not just this particular abhorrent boss; I didn't want *any* boss. I liked being in charge of my day and my future. I didn't adjust well to my disappointment and now refer to this period as "the dark ages."

It's relatively easy to stay motivated when the course is smooth and the finish line is within clear sight. On the other hand, when the path to an objective becomes difficult and muddled, dreams are often abandoned. I'm convinced that the key factor to achieving success or failure is whether you withstand the trials or walk away when adversity hits. I suppose that's the simple brilliance behind the old adage, "When the going gets tough, the tough get going." I knew what I wanted, and in spite of the odds being highly stacked against me, I chose to keep pushing and believing despite the turmoil it created.

Stress has consequences. As I would later learn during my ongoing MS research, I was living proof that times of anxiety can bring your disease out of dormancy. Stress impacts our bodies negatively no matter what condition or disease we're battling. From migraines to digestive issues to acne, stress makes them all worse. I sincerely believe if I hadn't experienced such angst at that time, my disease might have surfaced much later than when it did.

The irony reminds me of an Alanis Morissette hit. Remember 10,000 spoons when all you need is a knife? Isn't it ironic that when you're already feeling down and out, MS decides that it's the perfect time to rear its ugly head -- or in my case, shut down my right hand?

Once the initial shock of the resultant diagnosis subsided, I realized nothing about my life was immediately changing, so I jumped right back into my work mode. I was still a girl on a mission, and MS had yet to truly impact any of my abilities. MS or not, I wanted to achieve the top level with this company, and I was determined to make it happen.

In time, my boss at the part-time job gave me an ultimatum. He told me to close my "little candle thing" and go full-time for him "or else." Mr. S wanted to put me in charge of a new, bigger staffing business in a different location. To entice me, he took me to view the expanded office space and pitched the idea. At that moment, I knew what I had to do, and to this day, I thank him for making my choice abundantly clear. I made the obvious, albeit risky decision to quit that job and focus all of my energy and efforts into building *my* future, not his.

Being new to the area meant I was forced to be much more creative and aggressive about finding new networks of customers. I set challenging goals, made an effective plan and eventually turned my business into a large and very lucrative endeavor. Within a few years, I promoted to the highest level of the company with teams of consultants and leaders spanning the US and abroad. I learned invaluable goal setting, and interpersonal skills and, along the way discovered how to teach, encourage, and inspire others. What started from a last-minute candle party, turned into a 23-year-career with a wonderfully supportive direct sales company. Take that, MS!

My laser focus on the advancement potential of my business prevented me from getting stuck in the medical black hole that MS creates. Doctors, insurance companies, and medical bills are all riddled with time-consuming and defeating frustrations at every turn. Oh, if only I could get back all the wasted hours spent working to outsmart those evil automated phone systems. Designed to prevent us from actually talking to a live human, they serve as unofficial arrogant gatekeepers. After playing dodgeball through all the prompts, pressing the exact buttons in the right order to get to an actual person, and then clearly stating all of the correct information including birthdate, ID number, reason for contact, etc., I would invariably wait on multiple indefinite holds while being transferred to three different departments only to get disconnected and have to start the laborious process all over again.

It takes monumental fortitude to withstand these drawn out, torturous battles that most patients rarely win. However, the perilous journey would sometimes yield a desired end result. Little victories were celebrated when I successfully determined co-pays or found answers about basic things like eligibility for drugs or medical procedures.

Speaking of time invested in overcoming obstacles, how about trying to choose insurance options when none of them were affordable or met all of my needs with this pre-existing condition? So instead of being overwhelmed by all those frustrations early on, I chose to stick my head in the sand and live in denial about my disease as long as I possibly could.

I'm not promoting this repudiation of truth as a recommended coping mechanism. It may not be ideal, but like my mom, it's what I did to keep moving forward. Just as we all mourn differently after a tragic loss or devastating news, so too do we all play by different sets of rules after being hit with a dreaded diagnosis.

In the same way that a homeowner might delay the

necessary repair of an old roof until it rains, I chose to ignore MS. I certainly did my very best to hide it from others until MS made itself impossible to ignore, pouring down on me like a torrential spring thunderstorm.

When my hand function returned to normal, it was easy for me to disregard my presumed condition. Many of my fellow MS warriors are immediately burdened with debilitating symptoms that either temporarily or permanently turn their worlds upside down. I realize if that had been the case with my disease, denial wouldn't have been possible.

Later though, as my abilities began to slowly deteriorate, I still naively doubted the connection to MS. My bladder wasn't functioning well. The frequency, urgency and even hesitancy (yes, frustratingly, all three) increased, but I still didn't acknowledge that MS was the culprit. I started tripping over my own feet and losing coordination, but the changes were happening so gradually, I dismissed it as clumsiness. If elaborate justification was an art, then I was Van Gogh.

Once while attending an out-of-town conference, I was dressing for the day and as I stood to pull my pants on one leg while balancing on the other, I stumbled, almost in slow motion, to the ground. My roommate for the event saw the whole thing and was quite entertained by my embarrassing and ungraceful fall to the floor. I, too, realized how pitiful this whole scene looked and had to laugh at the absurdity. At the same time, I knew that my abilities seemed to be changing. [Sidenote:

31

I would never now attempt to balance on one leg while putting on pants. I have to be seated, or the aftermath will be ugly. Stumble, recalculate, adjust, and move on.]

Reluctantly, I began to acknowledge that my shifting anomalies weren't caused by a quirky bladder and a lack of coordination, but instead, this ridiculous disease. I didn't recognize the new body in which I now resided. The metamorphosis was so gradual, I almost unknowingly accommodated the changes in order to function. My gait widened, and I paid attention to every step. I avoided extreme heat and humidity and made sure to determine the location of all restrooms at any place I visited. I used the walls and surfaces around me for support and stability.

I certainly realized how fortunate I was to have my own business. Working a typical 8 to 5 grind wouldn't have been possible. I surely would have been forced to walk away from most other careers and file for disability. Also, from what I understand about that cumbersome process, there is no guarantee that disability would have been granted. How long would I have gone without income, and even if I had gotten the green light, how would I adjust to the reduced payments? Instead, my occupation allowed me to schedule my day according to my own needs and plans. Work, errands, hair appointments, or a needed rest can all be woven into each day at your own pace when you're self-employed.

As my symptoms progressed, I adjusted my personal level of business accordingly. I was doing fewer live events but became more intent on inspiring my teams utilizing the phone and other expanding technology. As my physical abilities declined, it was good for my soul to cheer others along as they accomplished their goals. I became a great encourager, often believing more in others than they believed in themselves. My work existence became centered around the idea that helping others achieve success ultimately benefits everyone! I was propelled by the quote from the late inspirational guru, Zig Ziglar: "You will get all you want in life if you help enough other people get what they want."

Most days included conference calls, one-on-ones or live trainings with my team who, for the most part, had no idea how much I was struggling to work through each day. Just getting from one side of my house to the other required logistical planning. Before leaving a room, I would make sure I had everything I needed because I didn't want to circle back and unnecessarily waste precious energy. Countless phone conversations happened alongside falls, doctor appointments, exercise, and fatigue, but I always managed to keep smiling and inspiring those around me, and many of my closest team members did a fabulous job of pitching in where I fell short. Helping mostly women make their own lives better was essentially a paycheck of the heart for me. Serving others had a positive impact on keeping my own hardships in perspective.

Ultimately, I think my body knew it was time for this change before my brain did. During the years when the routine of parties and trainings had become grueling, I kept fooling myself that I could handle it. It was becoming clear to me that my comfort zone was no longer comfortable.

CHAPTER THREE

Moving On

Always be a first-rate version of yourself instead of a second-rate
version of somebody else.
~ Judy Garland

As my changing abilities forced me to make adjustments to my career demands, another big life adjustment loomed. Years before when I promoted to the company's top level, we had built our dream home. That house was beautiful but entirely too big as it contained five+ bedrooms for two people who weren't even sure if children would be in their future. As my mobility became more challenged, navigating the three levels of this house became incredibly awkward. To make matters worse, some of those stairs going from the basement to the second floor were particularly steep.

Stairs are especially unwieldy for some of us with MS. When navigating flat, level ground your feet just need to move forward repeatedly. For me, that's already enough to require great concentration, so stairs take it to a whole new level. The multi-process messages from your brain to your feet need to fire much more quickly. I describe the feeling as trying to walk a straight line while being three sheets to the wind. However, in addition to being drunk, 'the line' is taking you through a path of peanut butter and the ground underneath is moving like the waves of the ocean. Meanwhile, you're experiencing some numbness, tingling, pain, fatigue and possibly a little vertigo all at the same time. The messages become more swift, complex and interdependent. Now you must lift your foot out of the peanut butter, balance momentarily on one foot while you brace against the crashing waves, move your hand to grab a higher spot on the handrail, keep your eyes on the next step, and then repeat the process with the other foot over and over.

Of course, what goes up must come down. Traversing down the stairs is even more difficult, so the method to my madness on many occasions was the same as many toddlers -- one step at a time on my behind. As a result of all this awkwardness, I plummeted down the stairs in that home many times though surprisingly never breaking my neck or ending up in a body cast.

Yes, my struggles were obviously pointing us to a change. We felt trapped in that giant house because we couldn't imagine all the work involved in selling a home and relocating. Of course the bigger the house, the more "stuff" you acquire which made the thought of packing and moving it all seem even more daunting and overwhelming. My poor husband knew that most of the work would fall on his already weary shoulders.

In addition, I mistakenly assumed that leaving my dream home meant I was succumbing to my dreadful disease. I had taken great pride in the design and decor of every inch of that house and believed I would never find another one that could bring me as much pride. How dare my MS force me to leave the home I loved! Looking back, I now realize that it was just the opposite. I was allowing, of all things, a structure made of wood and bricks to hold me back from an easier and more enjoyable life.

Once we concluded that downsizing (aka rightsizing) was logical and necessary, the process happened rather quickly. To lighten our load, we sold or donated some of the extra baggage we had acquired through the years. Who needs three patio sets and seven bar stools anyway? It was liberating to rid ourselves of the overabundance of furniture and pointless belongings more suited for a family of 10.

My beautifully appointed house sold within two days of being listed. As we hadn't yet discovered our next place, I put it out to the universe that our ideal one-level ranch would appear. We searched and viewed many possibilities but never felt sure about any until the day we stepped foot in the one we immediately purchased. Once again, I found that the universe always delivers!

We survived the painful moving process and now feel more settled and comfortable in our new residence than we ever did in the oversized dwelling we called home for 15 years. Now, the bedrooms and my workout room are all located on the main floor. No more stairs unless I navigate to the basement -- something I rarely do since everything I need is on the ground floor.

We are located in a more serene environment surrounded by parks and a nature preserve. To top it off, the house is stylishly updated and architecturally interesting with many soaring vaults and angles. The few undesirable features were quickly redesigned and modified to my specific tastes. This house just makes sense for us, and now we wonder why we waited so long.

After we moved and I realized how positive this colossal adjustment had been, I began to question the career in which I was also beginning to feel trapped. Was it truly practical for me to continue with a business I no longer felt physically capable of tackling? Like our decision to take a leap and move to a new home, I decided it might be time for a career move, too.

Holding in-home sales parties as well as spearheading and attending company events are the basics of this business. In my prime, I held an average of 4-5 parties a week. At one time, I spoke to audiences of up to 10,000 at week-long, company-wide national conferences. All these activities used to be enjoyable and energizing. Now they had become physically miserable for me. It was taking a toll. I was no longer capable of leading by example.

As the changes occurred, I also grew weary of being a has-been. I wasn't willing to continue training others to do things I could no longer do myself. So, with some sadness and relief, I confidently chose to take PartyLite's generous 10-year retirement package available to those who've reached the top level. I selected a fellow company leader to take the reins of my responsibilities and support my teams by being down in the trenches with them doing the job that had become nearly impossible for me. This organization was like my baby, and I wanted to ensure that my talented team members continued to flourish under their new leadership.

I can now relate to the aging father who still thinks of himself as a competent driver while barely avoiding accidents. If he continues in his denial of reality, his wife and/or children will ultimately have to take control of the car keys. Once I accepted this, I was ready. I made the decision.

Since I've stepped away from my former career, my wheels are turning again about what the future holds; I can't wait to see what the next chapter of my life brings. Over the years, helping colleagues improve their business has transitioned into helping others with MS. I've been honored to consult and offer support to many individuals with MS who were referred to me by a friend or acquaintance. I suppose I earned the reputation of MS Warrior as a result of my years of continuously moving forward in spite of this baffling condition doing its best to hold me back. Most frequently, I am asked to speak to someone dealing with shock and uncertainty after receiving their MS diagnosis. Then there are others who have been managing this disease for a long time and are always looking for common ground or suggestions from someone on a similar path. Either way, I value the responsibility I've been dealt.

I take great joy in sharing with others by giving educational empowerment talks to audiences made up of those coping with this disease as well as their friends and families. After these programs, it is a glorious feeling when some of my fellow MSers, who came there feeling scared and overwhelmed, tell me how much I have enlightened and encouraged them.

Even on those days when the disease is more challenging, I invariably feel better about my own situation when I impact others in a positive way. Lifting those around us ultimately elevates ourselves in the process. Yes, MS has taken a lot from me, but it's also given me an incredible opportunity to meet many heroes that I would never have crossed paths with otherwise. It's funny how a light of joy and satisfaction appears as the result of a desperate and sometimes hopeless situation.

Even though I can no longer walk unassisted without stumbling, I'm discovering new things at which I *can* excel. I anticipate facing continued challenges, failures and stumbles along the way. That's to be expected for anyone — especially during times of transition. However, I now spend less time lamenting the loss of who I used to be and instead choose to focus my limited energy on rising to become the best version of who I am today.

CHAPTER FOUR

Losing the Pride

Pride makes us artificial and humility makes us real.

~ Thomas Merton

Twenty-three years post diagnosis, my disease still feels like an enigma. After my initial useless hand symptom came and went, doctors predicted my course would likely be the most common MS type, "relapsing remitting." I was warned about ongoing clearly defined attacks, like the numb hand, followed by periods of partial or complete recovery, but that didn't happen. Those exacerbations would have confirmed my MS diagnosis, but I never suffered another relapse which meant, in my mind, I was beating this thing! I presumed, like the guy with hiccups, my hand peculiarity must have been a fluke. Because my disease stayed hidden early on, I mistakenly chose to ignore the "MS Patient" label I'd already seen typed on an insurance form. I didn't want that title, and if they were already making incorrect predictions, they were likely wrong about my diagnosis, too. In addition, my stubbornness meant that I would be the one to decide my future health, not a grumpy, old-school doctor putting unwanted labels next to my name. Swimming in a sea of medical uncertainty, that unwavering hopeful conviction was my life raft.

My continuing disdain for labels most certainly began as a child when I learned first hand how hard they are to shake. By 10 years of age, it was clear that I took after my dad's height and shot up faster than anyone in my class. In fourth grade, the elementary school basketball coach recruited me for his team even though the other players were in the upper grades. I was not only tall but was a thick, big boned kid which resulted in peers calling me fat. Very little is more traumatic to a young girl than being called "fat." To make matters worse, I acquired the nickname "Jolly Green Gina." Even after losing weight in college, I still saw that chunky girl's reflection in the mirror, and I continued purchasing clothes that were two sizes too big. Even though I'm the opposite of fat now, the "fat girl" moniker still sometimes toys with my mind.

Because I'd been anxious to drop the MS label, I'd gone to another neurologist for a second opinion. The second opinion led to confusion that only fueled my denial. Around this time, MS related brochures started mysteriously arriving in the mail.

Who knew about this whole thing anyway? I was keeping it quiet after all. Some of the pamphlets encouraged me to attend an upcoming MS support group meeting. Even though I wasn't interested in fitting into this group, I was curious. Maybe I'd meet others who understood the unsure diagnoses I'd received. I decided to try one. I don't remember where the event was held at or even what the space looked like, but I'll never forget how it made me feel. As I walked into a room full of people who looked very different than me, my heart sank. Was this what I had to look forward to? I didn't listen to much of what they said because I couldn't get beyond their support devices scattered around the room. There were canes leaning against walls, walkers at the hands of their owners, and wheelchairs holding two of the people. A support group specifically geared toward newly diagnosed patients would have been the right choice at that time, but those events weren't available in my area back then. These people were struggling with things I couldn't even comprehend: Vision problems, confusion, pain, gait issues, fatigue, needles. I felt out of place and didn't appreciate the harsh reminder of the depressing diagnosis I'd been thus far attempting to ignore. They discussed other things besides their conditions, but I don't remember anything else. I think they invited me back, and while I probably thanked them for welcoming me, once I escaped, I vowed never to return. Those devices wouldn't be in my future. I could run. I could jump. I felt invincible. I would fight harder to stay fit and strong, avoiding my neurologist like the plague. They could slap that

MS label on someone else -- not me! Just like "fat girl," I didn't need that one hanging around either.

Of course my avoidance of labels, support groups, and neurologists didn't change what was happening to my brain and spinal cord. As the years passed, I continued to be "reminded" of old Dr. B's words. Things started going wrong and kept deteriorating. Eventually and unwillingly, I had to accept the original diagnosis.

I didn't have a series of exacerbations as predicted. Instead, my MonSter stayed hidden for many years and eventually crept in and seized basic abilities right from under me. Now it's likely transitioning to a "secondary progressive" stage which is characterized by a gradual but sporadic worsening of those symptoms. Currently, I've been at a plateau for several years dealing with the same lost abilities with which I've grown "comfortably" familiar.

On the bright side, despite whatever subtype of MS I have, annual MRIs show I haven't had a new lesion in years. So far, my impacted abilities are essentially the same ones I've been dealing with and adjusting to for several years and will hopefully be the only issues I have forever. They have gotten slightly worse over the past few years because of what my doctor calls "senescence" of those old plaques. In other words, except for wine and wisdom, most things -- including my well-ripened lesions -- don't improve with age. That might not seem like a positive scenario to most people, but to someone who dreads new types of disease symptoms, the familiarity of my current condition is reassuring. Although my current MS limitations are a constant battle, at least I know what I'm up against and can focus on improving the adaptations I've been making for many years.

As a result of the long-term adjustments, I've become a master of discovering new ways to get things done. Adjustment should be my middle name. For example, with a slight tremor in both hands and impaired fine motor skills, writing a note or applying mascara have become daunting tasks. Careful concentration and encouraging self-talk help such as, "Steady. Take your time. No rush. You've got this." are crucial. With tedious determination, those tasks can be accomplished. Thank goodness, as mascara is one of life's little necessities.

However, independent adaptation and positive reinforcement can only take you so far. Sometimes help is needed, and unfortunately, it took me quite a while to accept it. Now, at this point in my MS progression, I know my life would be impossible without the support of mobility devices. So why did I wait so long? To be perfectly honest, fear, vanity, ego, and maybe some headstrong pride prevented me from using these helpful devices for many years. I've always taken great pride in my appearance and these contraptions were not my idea of stylish "accessorizing." My one visit to the support group meeting certainly didn't help either.

For me, concern over appearance began in my early childhood. From the age of 2 until first grade, I was groomed and adorably outfitted by a daytime housekeeper/nanny named Tish. My parents employed her for several years to keep our home functioning smoothly while they were immersed each day in running their many businesses. She was quirky, loving, and attentive, and I considered her like a third grandmother. Her goals each day were to keep every inch of our house tidy and to primp me like her own personal baby doll. She styled my hair in finger-curled ringlet pigtails and dressed me to the nines in hand-made, color-coordinated two piece outfits. In a *Brady Bunch* analogy, she was the Alice to my Cindy. The plaid polyester pants with coordinating button-up smocks were my favorite. As the baby of the family, I coveted the attention and relished being the apple of Tish's eye.

Through the years, she enjoyed taking me to photo shoots that resulted in many 8x10 glossies. She also coached me to sing and perform for groups at nursing homes and churches as she mouthed the words from the front row, lest I forget the lyrics. My older sisters didn't receive Tish's doting attention. They wore unmatched clothes, got dirty, and did their own thing. I joined them on the weekends when my parents were running the show, but Monday through Friday, I was kept unsoiled and well-polished. Naturally, my sisters attribute Tish's "Gina-obsession" with my lifelong attention to my external presentation.

In spite of the unpredictability of MS, I am comforted by always showing my best self. Since I no longer have Tish fixing my hair, salon blowouts are my weakness. My futile attempts to wash, dry, and style leave me feeling exhausted. In my defense, I do have highly challenging hair. It's a combination of wild frizz and coarse random curls which make it nearly impossible to tame. Once I entered first grade, Tish didn't arrive at our home until after I left for school. Without Tish, I had no idea what to do with my willful mane and was envious of classmates who could simply wash and go. I often resembled a jungle child fending for herself in the wild alongside the tigers and lions. My dad lovingly called me "Big Hair" which was yet another label that fueled my hair frustration and subsequent hair hang-up. As a result, I now leave it to the professionals and the miraculous things they can do with a hair dryer as often as possible. The contrast is quite obvious when I choose to "fix" it myself. And guess what? I'm also a regular at the nail salon for professional manis and pedis, too.

One might argue this kind of vanity is a subconscious attempt to combat the image of being dependent on utilitarian mobility devices. Or maybe I'm aiming to hide the disease behind my appearance. Actually, MS or not, this is just who I am. Perhaps it's Tish-inspired, but those blowouts, manis, and pedis simply make me feel good. As I write today, my nails are a glistening cobalt blue and yesterday's blowout still looks amazing, so when I catch a glimpse of either one, I smile.

I once identified with Billy Crystal and his "Fernando's Hideaway" character from *Saturday Night Live* who regularly professed in his Argentinian accent, "Dah-ling, you look mah-velous. It's better to look good than to feel good." As I've matured, however, I now strongly disagree with Fernando. Currently, if I was forced to choose between both options, I would much rather *feel* good. However, I still feel better when I look my best and prefer to have people look at *me* first instead of my device/disease. It's fun to shatter the "chronic disease" image in most people's minds. As with most "invisible" medical conditions, when people meet me for the first time they can't believe I have MS. How could someone who looks so put together and healthy have a deteriorating disease of the central nervous system? It's only when they see me walk or use a device that it becomes clear I'm afflicted with something. Ah, the dueling perceptions of living with an invisible disease!

Hence part of the reason why, even though I needed them, I didn't want anything to do with mobility devices. I was overly concerned with the image of using a cane. What would people think? If only I could recapture the precious energy wasted on that pointless and limiting paranoia. I now remind myself daily that it's none of my business what people think. As my wise son puts it, "Who cares what they think anyway?" While this is true, I prefer to not appear drunk at 10:00am. When I walk unassisted, one might rightly assume I've had a few too many margaritas. Finally, after dealing with too many strangers inquiring if I was "ok", I reluctantly decided to use the cane...but *only* in certain situations -- my first baby steps toward help.

Before this, I relied on things like chairs and walls for balance. I became an expert furniture and wall-walker. The downfall of this style of maneuvering is that when I leaned on something unstable or not positioned as expected, I would go down with a BANG. My likelihood of falling increased dramatically because of foolish pride and vanity. Spray tans became my summer response to mask bruise-covered arms and legs -- another tool of denial and disguise.

Here is a prime example of the kind of situations I found myself in before the cane: we were enjoying some pooltime on a family spring-break vacation to Florida. As usual, I needed to find a restroom very quickly. With MS, I'm not usually given much warning because the message from my bladder to my brain travels a disrupted irregular pathway. By the time I realize what's happening, it's already panic time. I sometimes imagine MS as a cruel and demented witch who sadistically cursed me with a spastic and neurogenic bladder as well as defective legs that can't move quickly enough to reach a bathroom in time. I've been traumatized and embarrassed by enough "accidents" that I regularly overcompensate to ensure it doesn't happen again.

Anyway, my husband and son were splashing way down

at the other end of the pool, so my mission was clear. I would make a beeline to the restroom unassisted and on my own. A group of jolly vacationers gathered for cocktail-hour by the pool watched as I zigzagged and bounced like a pinball between the pool chairs and the fencing in my wide-brimmed sun hat and sarong. With a sweet Southern twang, a concerned woman asked, "Do you need some help, sweetie? It looks like you've had a little too much fun in the sun, if you know what I mean," prompting the entire group to erupt into raucous laughter. There was simply no time to acknowledge them or explain my plight, so I pushed on determinedly, albeit haphazardly, weaving to and fro. My ignoring them and forging ahead caused the cocktail crowd to laugh even harder. Little did they know that alcohol is virtually off limits for me. Both alcohol and caffeine wreak havoc on my bladder which means Long Island Iced Teas would be the ultimate drink disaster. Perhaps if I'd at least had a cane in hand, the pool party crew might have cut me a little slack.

When I finally picked up a cane, it was better than nothing, but I used it only as a prop. At least with a cane in hand, I reasoned that observers wouldn't automatically wonder about how much alcohol I'd consumed. The problem is that a cane doesn't keep me moving in a straight line. Now the image shifted to an inebriated woman with a cane which seemed even more pitiful. Furthermore, a cane does not prevent me or a drunk person from stumbling and crashing to the ground. I've since learned that many savvy MS warriors flash a postcard that simply states. "I'm not drunk. I have MS." Brilliant!

My neurologist couldn't convince me to try any other devices, so instead she scheduled a physical therapy session to teach me the proper use of a cane. Who knew there were rules of cane usage? She explained that the physical therapist (PT) specialized in treating people with MS, so I begrudgingly agreed to the appointment. After asking questions and taking extensive notes, the PT asked me to walk around the little indoor track with my cane. After one lap evaluating my awkward cane cadence, I was quite surprised when the therapist retrieved a walker from a storage room. She encouraged me to be open minded and give it a shot. I confidently traipsed around the track and reported feeling confident and sure footed! It was just like using a shopping cart, but I wasn't ready to go there. I didn't know another woman in her forties who was using a walker. I was barely okay with the idea of a cane, so there was no way I was using a walker!

As I shed a couple tears, the kind 30-something therapist seemed to understand and despite her concern about me leaving with only the quasi-helpful cane, she did convince me to at least acquire a handicapped parking placard. This was a safety precaution that ended up changing my world. I had become quite the highly-competitive parker, driving around a parking lot for 15 minutes or more, searching for the absolute best parking spot I could find. I would stalk shoppers with packages in hand as they headed to their cars in hopes I could nab a front row spot as they left. Even though I was concerned about the picture of a healthy looking person who may be fraudulently hijacking a handicapped spot, the placard was a helpful modification, so I adjusted.

I was actually approached once by an overly-diligent mall cop who wondered why I was parking in a handicapped spot. He looked skeptical when I stated, "My legs don't work so well because I have MS." It briefly crossed my mind to take an intentional pavement face plant just to rub his nose in the fact that he was being a shortsighted heel. I was learning that as long as I had my cane prop, I could avoid stares and questions from such curious skeptics.

While this adjustment definitely helped in parking lots, it didn't prevent injuries of my toes, ankles, knees, elbows, ribs, and most recently an upper eyelid that led to a black eye a la Rocky Balboa. None of those falls happened in parking lots, but instead, resulted from mishaps at home. After I'd experienced pain, stitches, surgeries, and orthopedic boots, I was closer to acknowledging that if I could reduce the number of ER visits, that alone might be worth swallowing my pride and utilizing some mobility devices.

It's not a good sign when you see your orthopedist so often that you know what's happening in his personal life. "So the last time I was here you were heading to a vacation in

California. How was it?" A doctor's office is not exactly the kind of place that you want to visit so often that, like the tv show *Cheers'* theme song, "...everybody knows your name, and they're always glad you came."

I vividly remember the agony that ensued while visiting my favorite deli in a small local Italian grocery store/cafe when I was still boycotting mobility assistance. I'd already stocked up on bags of groceries at a big chain grocery store next door but still needed sandwich meat for that week's lunches. Once I arrived at the deli counter, I could see they were especially busy, so I grabbed a number and waited my turn. I was number 48, and they had just called 37. After a string of indecisive customers who were thoughtfully sampling multiple meat and cheese varieties, I realized I needed a trip to the restroom. It was, of course, in the back of the store. The little family-run business had recently eliminated the use of shopping carts in an attempt, I suppose, to shift their image to more of a restaurant than market. So, with no cart for support, I looked past the deli, the shelves of groceries, and the dining area to the back wall where the restroom was located, wondering how I would ever make it there unsupported. It looked as daunting as if I were a contestant on *American Ninja Warrior* forced to traverse a narrow balance beam while precariously dodging various flying obstacles. I leaned on everything in my path for stability -- the olive bar, several chair backs and tabletops, the wine display and fountain drink station -- and miraculously made it just as my legs were beginning to wobble. Victory was mine! However, when I exited the restroom, my elation was short-lived. I looked beyond the deli counter through the clear glass storefront to my car in the handicapped spot. It might as well have been a 10-mile hike, and in my weary state, I had absolutely no idea how I would transport myself there with legs that were completely shot. Defeated and alone, I ungracefully fell into one of the cafe booths immediately outside the restroom. I would station myself there long enough for my legs to hopefully "recharge" so I could eventually make it to my car.

A group of ladies who were there enjoying a girls' lunch happened to notice me obviously looking forlorn. They'd probably seen me stumble to the restroom and then collapse into the booth. One of them stood up, and before I knew it, was sitting directly across from me in the booth where I was now stranded. She placed her hand on top of mine and asked if I was okay. I was on the verge of tears and attempting to distract myself by fiddling with my phone. I was surprised that my struggle was so obvious to others, yet her kindness brought my emotion to the surface. I tried to explain through now gushing tears that I had MS and had gotten through the entire store but didn't know how I would make it back to the deli counter and then to my car. She told me that she was a nurse, and she understood my condition. She got up and came around to my side of the booth to give me a big hug that told me she really did understand! She swiftly fetched me a cup of water and some tissues and asked more questions.

When had I been diagnosed? Was I on my own that day? Did I have a cane or walker? Even though she was a complete stranger, I opened up about my whole story. She asked if she could do anything to help me return back to the deli counter and then to my car? I said yes, there was one thing. While I had been stuck there feeling sorry for myself I'd also been eyeing a lone shopping cart that was maybe 20 feet away. I looked toward it longingly and explained that it was obviously being used by employees to transport inventory from the back. It was full of various tomato sauces and uncooked pasta waiting to be placed on shelves. I was confident that if I could just grab the handle of that cart for support, I could make it back to the deli counter and then to my car. She immediately stood up, grabbed the cart, and quickly delivered it to me. I was as ecstatic as if she had just handed me the keys to a vault full of gold bars. I hugged her again and thanked her profusely. I made it to the deli counter and got the pound of stupid maple turkey which had originally inspired this whole mess! After I paid the cashier, that kind-hearted soul met me at the door and allowed me to grab her arm for support as we walked to my car. I was so full of gratitude at that point, I gave her a third hug. I don't know who she was and never asked her name, but I believe she was placed there to impact my life that day. I'll never forget her. She reinforced the truth in what my dad had always said: "This world is full of good people!"

After a few more traumatic experiences like that, I became very selective about leaving the house. If it's not an immediate necessity, it could wait. I certainly learned the hard way about my one-stop limit. If I tackled one location, I wouldn't plan on another until the next day. I know that many MSers can relate. When you take my particular MS recipe of poor balance and leg weakness and combine it with a pinch of spasticity, numbness, and tingling followed by a dash of fatigue and neurological back pain, and a generous helping of urinary frequency/urgency, home becomes a precious sanctuary. Fortunately, I've embraced online shopping and have become skilled at finding exactly what I want/need with a couple clicks. I'm particularly appreciative of stores that deliver directly to your door or allow you to order online but have designated pick-up areas where staff load items directly into your car. Even if you don't have mobility issues, this type of shopping is a time and money saver. An added bonus is that you completely avoid those alluring impulse aisles which were the bane of my shopping existence pre MS. No longer will I waste my precious energy acquiring dish soap and toilet paper for my family. Thank you, technology!

As my erratic bladder was the indirect cause of these disasters, I was prescribed several drug remedies over the years. None of them worked, so I was referred to a urogynecologist who injected $8,000 worth of botox into my bladder every few months. It helped a little. Before each session, I always asked the doctor if he could save a bit for my eyes, but no luck so far. I've learned that the muscles around my bladder are extra strong and overdeveloped. While viewing my bladder muscles on a little TV during the botox procedure, one doc described them as thick and strong "like tree trunks." Apparently, in an attempt to compensate for the delayed messages, they've actually strengthened, leaving me with a spastic bladder that overreacts and goes into a squeezing and convulsing frenzy at the slightest suggestion of a needed bathroom visit. Interesting that the muscles I've never exercised in the gym have become my strongest and most well developed of all. Yes, I'm proud to have a buff bladder!

Despite the Italian market debacle, I was still a "selective" mobility device user. Call me a slow learner. If I felt strong and stable on a certain day, I might shortsightedly decide to skip the support. On a particularly confident day a couple years ago, I decided to visit a department store in search of a new outfit for an upcoming event. This wasn't the type of store with ride-on carts for its physically-challenged shoppers, and I mistakenly thought I could make it using a small, unstable push cart for stability. To be clear, even if they'd had a ride-on device, I probably wouldn't have used it for fear of being seen by someone I knew.

I browsed the racks engrossed in my search. I wasn't even planning to try on the clothes that looked promising as that would definitely take too much energy. I'm a seasoned shopper and can usually decipher whether an outfit will work based on the cut, style, and fabric. If I chose well, I also wouldn't need to venture back to return anything. I was on a roll.

Thoroughly absorbed in my shopping bubble and forgetting all about MS, it hit. I needed to find a bathroom and quickly. Here we go again! I knew better than this. How had I gotten so caught up in shopping that I hadn't considered the inevitable challenges and limitations that constantly plague me? With my tree trunk bladder muscles spasming, weary legs objecting and a few rest-stops along the way, I barely made it all the way to the restroom in the back of the store. However, the relief was fleeting when I exited the restroom and realized the overwhelming challenge ahead of me. With my overcooked spaghetti-like legs maneuvering through the crashing waves and peanut butter, how could I possibly transport myself to the front of the store, find a register, and pay for my new stylish blouse? I was so enthralled in my search for one of the trendy cold-shoulder tops that I hadn't even had time to search for any bottoms. Considering my current situation, I knew that I could eventually make it back to my car but waiting in line at a register looked doubtful.

As the clock ticked, my mind raced with all I still needed to accomplish before my son got off the bus that afternoon. Even so, all I could do was sit outside the bathroom doors by the water fountain on a bench designed for patiently waiting spouses. I was stranded again. My legs are like a cell phone battery. When they run out of charge, the only remedy is to sit and wait for them to recharge. If I can get them up to 20%, they will work at least temporarily. The ideal situation is to charge them all the way up to 100%, but I didn't have that kind of time. I gave up on the new outfit and decided I could just find something in my own closet anyway. I reluctantly laid the cute blouse on the bench. Now on top of everything else, I was stooping to the loser retail customer level by leaving inventory in weird places. I'd worked in retail years ago and knew how maddening that was for the employees.

While stuck at my leg-charging station, my mind wandered to the spoons. I'd recently learned from a fellow MSer, Chadd, about the Spoon Theory and knew that my spoons were all used up for the day. This idea, created by lupus sufferer Christine Miserandino, equates spoons to energy levels in a person with a disability or chronic illness.[1] I imagined that everybody scurrying past the bench had purses and shopping carts overflowing with spoons. My spoon supply, however, was completely depleted. While my husband and son start each day with bunches of spoons, I only start with a few and when they're gone, they're gone. Oh, what I would have given right then for just a few of Alanis Morissette's 10,000 spoons.

I decided to call my husband. Only he would understand the difficulty of my miserable predicament. I had barely

---

1   https://butyoudontlooksick.com/articles/written-by-christine/the-spoon-theory/

explained the sad series of events before he quickly said he would make the 45 minute drive from work to rescue me. I told him that my lack of planning shouldn't inconvenience his day, and besides, in 45 minutes my legs would likely be ready to make the trek. Even though I refused his help, hearing his concern and worry at such a vulnerable moment was a relief. After enough time passed, I slowly, painfully, and empty-handedly made it back to my car. I celebrated when I got in, vowing to never find myself stuck in that helpless situation again. I had to accept that my "battery" didn't have the life it once had.

I remember fondly those day-long shopping trips to the mall. I could mindlessly navigate from one end to the other carrying several packages and covering multiple floors and fitting rooms for hours on end. Nowadays with mobility challenges, the mall is a complete danger zone. Fortunately, I've matured so I no longer have a burning desire to hang out at the mall like I once did. Shopping without a specific purpose is now a luxury I can't justify. I'd rather save my energy for more important pursuits. But, it's nice to know if I need to, I can. When MSers start missing out on activities or events because of our limited spoon condition, we know it's time to let the devices do what they are designed to do: assist and open our worlds. Mobility aids are a must no matter how strong we feel or unattractive they look.

Due to the amount of planning required for a simple

trip to the supermarket followed by the overwhelming fatigue, MSers often become trapped in their homes. It's safer there. We know where things are, including the restroom, and how to maneuver to get there. When we get tired, we can take a break. We don't have to get our mobility tools charged and loaded in the car, and we don't have to risk paying the price with more fatigue later. This is the point where our worlds begin to shrink making MS a lonely and isolating plight. On top of the loneliness, not many people understand the disease. I used to struggle for words to answer inevitable questions from those curious types who would ask what was wrong with me. Had I undergone surgery recently? Was I recovering from a broken bone or a sprained ankle? At first, I would answer, "Yep, I just keep plugging along and eventually I get there." I suppose it was a lie of omission, but at the time, I just thought it was easier. As I became more experienced, I tweaked my answer a bit and became comfortable saying, "No I actually have multiple sclerosis, and my legs don't cooperate." I've now learned it's important to be honest and open and to surround myself with people who want to understand what I deal with on a daily basis. Rather than masquerading as something I'm not, I choose to build awareness to inform those who might otherwise misunderstand this confounding disease.

My most preferred supportive device is still my husband's strong arm. He holds it up, cocked and held tight at a 90 degree angle. It's reminiscent of the day he escorted me down the aisle after we exchanged vows so many years ago. When we walk together, he senses when I start to stumble, slowing down while I grab on tighter, all the while preparing to catch me if I fall. I feel completely safe, supported, and proud to hang onto this hunky guy. The problem with my chosen support tool, however, is that its owner has a life and isn't always available at my beck and call. Additionally, waiting for my husband's assistance does not maintain my "hear me roar" independence. So yes, I was learning to accept that using a mechanical device or two brings me more opportunity and freedom.

CHAPTER FIVE

Building a Toolbox

Faith is taking the first step, even when you don't see the whole staircase.

~ Martin Luther King, Jr.

A few years ago, we visited a medical supply store. We were in the market for a wheelchair which would allow our little family to visit places that required extensive walking. In St.Louis, we have a wonderful children's museum, zoo, and science center, and I was disappointed that these great venues had become off limits. As my husband and son helped me choose the right wheelchair, I fought back tears while comparing the features of each one. Ever since my initial diagnosis years before, I dreaded the idea of being confined to a wheelchair. Here I was now, smack dab in the middle of a shopping trip for exactly that.

While I selected the size and color, my observant son reassured me with his wisdom saying, "Mom, just think of all the possibilities this chair opens up! We can go places and do things that we haven't been able to. We should call this the "Possibilities Chair!" And so it was. My Possibilities Chair has come in handy countless times. Sometimes it's easier to maneuver a chair than a walker or scooter, so I have all three.

Of all the mobility devices I now own, the one most difficult to mentally accept is the most valuable to me -- the walker. When my son was a baby, I loved pushing him for long walks in a stroller. We would leave our neighborhood and go in all directions, trekking a few miles as he dozed. I was sad when he outgrew his stroller and selfishly tried to confine him to one longer than he wanted. No wonder his favorite thing to do now is run; I don't think he's sat down since! As our long walks became more difficult, I realized I wouldn't be able to go very far at all without pushing the stroller. I needed the support to help me march forward in a straight line. Without it, I was all zig-zag and stumbles. For this same reason, I grew to love shopping carts. Like a stroller, they allowed me to look like everyone else while providing the support I needed. Basically, I was essentially using a walker disguised as something else. Unfortunately, shopping carts weren't prevalent in my neighborhood, so when the stroller became obsolete, I was stuck in the house.

Like most, I associated walkers with nursing homes and the elderly. My mom was forced into nursing home rehab after breaking her hip at 80-years-old. Once she was past the initial trauma of the situation, she was forced to rely on a walker and eventually a wheelchair. When she complained about using them, I gave her little sympathy about needing the helpful aids. I remember responding to her complaints saying, "Mom you're 80! Imagine how you would have felt using a walker or wheelchair at my age. When you were in your 40s, you could have run circles around me. You're going to heal and get past this; I won't." I wasn't trying to be heartless to my mother but instead was attempting to reinforce what I thought was the temporary nature of her situation. Maybe I should have been more sensitive. This journey has been gradual for me. For her, like many seniors, it happened after one disastrous fall.

Now that I've finally accepted them, one of my three walkers is with me all the time. I use one to navigate on the main floor of my house. I have another on the lower level so that when I venture downstairs, it's waiting for me there, and my third one is always in the backseat of my car. It's lightweight and easily collapsible like an umbrella stroller so it's perfect for on-the-go. Now that I appreciate the walker's purpose, I would much rather walk short distances without injury and get some exercise rather than ride everywhere on a scooter or wheelchair. Of course, occasionally I'm caught off guard by comments from clueless strangers. Recently while entering a restaurant, a chatty lady watching me push the walker to the entrance said, "You look too young for that!" I considered responding with a simple explanation about the realities of MS and the typical age of diagnosis for those of us dealing with it, but instead, flashed a big grin and said, "Thanks...I guess" and kept moving. Spreading awareness can be noble, but sometimes dealing with people's ignorance is just tiring.

The most recent addition to my device toolbox is a mobility scooter. Admittedly, I had to mentally adjust to this one, too. I couldn't shake the image of George Costanza's *Seinfeld* character looking comical on the Little Rascal scooter while faking his disability in order to keep the spacious handicap accessible bathroom at a new job. I didn't want to be perceived as a fraud, like him. It's not that I can't walk; I just can't go very far. However, I've now accepted the scooter's leg saving value. It gives me freedom that the wheelchair simply can't. In a wheelchair, I lost the sense of control one has when walking upright. Also, when in a wheelchair, I essentially became nearly invisible to everyone I passed. It's the oddest thing but most people don't know what to say to someone in a wheelchair. I'm only a couple feet lower than they are, but it's as if the chair magically renders me either invisible or incapable of thought. I challenge anyone to get down to their level, make eye contact with, and ask the next person they see in a wheelchair this question, "Hey there, how are you doing today?" They will probably appreciate being acknowledged.

With a scooter, I have the independence of my own wheels. I'm in charge of where I'm going instead of relying on someone else to push me. It comes apart in four pieces and is easily transported in the back of my SUV. However, in spite of my basic five and eight pound weight lifting routine, I'm not coordinated or strong enough to balance, lift, and assemble the heavy parts by myself which means that the scooter doesn't give me full autonomy. I'm currently toying with the idea of adding a lift device on the rear of my car. I'm not there yet, but maybe that will be my next baby step. In the meantime, the scooter has been exceptionally useful for attending my son's baseball games.

Imagine the anxiety when you realize you need to make it to the farthest field from the parking lot. After wondering how you will get there, the fear rises to a new level when you contemplate transporting yourself from the bleachers to the restroom in a timely fashion as your hulk-like bladder walls squeeze away. Before the scooter, and despite knowing how unhealthy it was, I would prepare for such situations by purposely dehydrating myself. I was like a camel; if I had an evening commitment, I drank my entire day's worth of water in the morning so I could start my dehydration process in the afternoon. I did what I had to. Now I can zip past everyone else at the ballpark in record time thanks to the jackrabbit speed setting on my trusty scooter. I adore watching my son play ball so this accommodation has been especially worthwhile.

When dealing with a difficult situation, why not have the best options available? Great photographers often keep numerous cameras and lenses on hand depending on the shoot, and skilled carpenters pack their boxes full of a variety of tools to tackle a myriad of tasks, so it's fitting that a person with mobility issues should arm herself with a variety of resources to make life easier and more accessible.

Some of my required accommodations are less device and more a combination of awareness, preparation, and proactiveness. Lack of balance causes many an obscure and somewhat amusing challenge. Due to lesions and possible cell death in my cerebellum that affect my vestibular system, vision is the only tool I have to maintain balance. If I close my eyes or if I'm in a completely dark room and not stabilizing myself with something, I can drop to the ground quicker than a box of rocks.

Neurologists give a test called Romberg's Sign to determine neurological function relating to balance. The patient is asked to stand with feet together looking forward and then told to -- this is the part that gets me -- close his/her eyes. The doctor then looks for swaying or loss of balance. Needless to say, this is definitely a test I fail every time. It's also the same test a police officer gives to a suspected intoxicated driver. Fortunately, since I drive while seated and with my eyes open, I'm not like a drunk person on the road. This neurological anomaly, however, does deliver a few less obvious safety issues.

Since it's physically impossible to keep your eyes open when you sneeze, this presents me with a particularly interesting conundrum. When I feel a sneeze brewing, I better sit down or lean against the wall or there will be trouble. While it sounds rather comical, I've experienced a few ugly sneeze-related falls and injuries. When you sneeze and end up on the floor, vanity becomes the least of your concerns.

Washing one's hair hardly seems like a potential hazard. Most of us close our eyes when water rushes over our heads. If I'm not securely hanging onto the shower grab bar when eyes are closed, there will be trouble. I thought this particular crisis would be averted by the extensive master bathroom remodel in our new home. With its sleek grey and white design complete with a zero entry tile shower, built-in seat and grab bars galore, it rivals many of the swanky bathrooms at five star hotels I've visited over the years on business. In spite of all the safety measures, however, just one slippery shampoo grip on the grab bar resulted in a crash to the floor -- but not before striking and bursting my eyelid on the shower bench. One inch lower, and it would have been much worse. Upon hearing the crash followed by my anguished scream, my husband rushed in to find me crumpled on the shower floor, covered in blood. It was probably eerily reminiscent of the infamous *Psycho* shower scene. As usual, Scott came to my rescue, picked me up and, not always embracing the glass half-full attitude like me, decided he would start wrapping me in bubble wrap before I shower.

While it actually sounds a little kinky, I don't think I would get very clean with all the plastic. Instead, we compromised with me agreeing to actually use the very stable built-in shower seat to wash my hair instead of cracking open my head. This experience also further justified the expense of my "very safe" salon blowouts!

Even though my disease is invisible, the mobility devices I've finally accepted are not. I fought them because I didn't want to appear weak. Now I've learned these helpers in fact, allow me to be stronger. I can independently accomplish more with less risk of a debilitating injury. It's like playing on a sports team that has an injured player. Just as the rest of the team is required to pick up the slack, so does Scott in our family when I'm laid up after a fall. Scott takes on a new level of activity to compensate for his teammate who's officially on the DL. For years, my loving husband strongly encouraged me to embrace the support while I stubbornly fought it. It took many stumbles before I finally got out of my own way and figured that out. I had to learn that I need to lean on support to make me stronger while being safely independent. Now I'm committed to building the strongest toolbox possible to continue rising farther than I ever imagined! I'm grateful to have finally figured out that no one can do life unsupported -- not even me.

Ego isolates and divides us. I was so busy trying to hide my disease that I didn't realize I was closing myself off to the world. When I began sharing my true self and connecting with people through the vulnerabilities that we all have, it was pretty remarkable. It was as if my world opened up and started giving me the most delightful gifts. Once I stopped hiding and fully embraced the devices, I felt joy and was rejuvenated by letting others in. I experienced acts of kindness from complete strangers and made new friendships because of my authenticity, and for that, I've finally arrived at a place where I'm grateful for what MS has given me.

CHAPTER SIX

Getting Behind the Wheel

You must take personal responsibility. You cannot change the
circumstances, the seasons, or the wind, but you can
change yourself.
~ Jim Rohn

This disease creates helplessness as we lose control of basic physical abilities. If I would have peered into a crystal ball 30 years ago and saw the limits I face today, I would have been devastated. My diminished abilities have delivered a one-two punch to some of my favorite activities and basic life expectations. Out of nowhere, it swooped into my world with its cruel intentions, and in true *Invasion of the Body Snatchers* style, slowly attacked my physical capabilities from within. Post diagnosis, I attempted to hide for many years from my condition, but MS wouldn't allow me to do so forever.

When my son was about two-and-a-half years old and still in the stroller, I suspected the changes I was experiencing were MS related. I was tripping on my own feet, falling down and had unsuccessfully tried every bladder med on the market. After approximately 12 years ignoring my disease, I had developed new lesions. When I heard my doctor's report after an MRI, I felt violated as if the ugly war-ravaged MonSter had been covertly invading and sabotaging my body while allowing me to believe I had outplayed the demon. At the same time, I was frustrated with myself for letting my disease go untreated all those years. If I had begun a therapy immediately upon diagnosis, perhaps I could have kept the MonSter at bay so that it wouldn't have woven those patchy lesions around my brain and spinal cord. Currently, there are more than 14 disease modifying drugs (DMD's) administered in several different methods. None of them are a cure or will eliminate the disease but offer a "cross-your-fingers" hope that new lesions won't form. Studies show that disease progression is slower when receiving long term disease-modifying drug treatment. I recently heard a neurologist speak at an MS event about why it's imperative to begin a DMD immediately after diagnosis. She explained that for every year without an available therapy, you might later expect a 5% increase in your level of disability. Since I had delayed treatment 12 years, I estimated I was about 60% further declined in my MS progression. My husband and mom both repeatedly offered some solace with a quote shared by Scott's Grandpa Stines. "If ifs and buts were candy and nuts, we'd all have a Merry Christmas." While I can't change the past, I can learn from it and use it to help others. Basically, live and learn.

When I was diagnosed, there were only three possible DMD's available to hopefully slow progression of MS, but I was unwilling to consider taking the intrusive interferon drugs because of their lengthy lists of side effects. Besides, my master plan was to ignore my diagnosis.

Like my mom, I've never been shy about quizzing doctors for their honest opinions, so when things really started to progress, I asked my neurologist one simple question: If her daughter had MS, would she advise her to do the dreaded shots? The framed photos of her high-achieving girls were displayed proudly among her own diplomas and certificates. When the doc answered that she would definitely encourage her daughter to try anything FDA-approved to slow the progression, I knew I literally had to give it "a shot."

I chose the DMD with the least frequent dosing schedule. A nurse trained me how to inject myself once a week with a long needle that I hoped contained a helpful drug into the muscle of my leg. After insurance picked up most of the tab for this $6,000 per month treatment, we were responsible for

a $452 monthly co-pay. After just paying a $3,200 MRI bill the
week before, we dreaded our new expense. We could certainly
think of many more exciting ways to spend hundreds of dollars
a month rather than for "possible flu-like symptoms."

When the nurse sent me home with my new bright red
Sharps container, I wondered what in the world I had agreed to.
I'd seen those red boxes covered in hazardous waste stickers in
medical offices, but I never imagined owning one myself. I didn't
display it as in a doctor's office but instead kept it tucked away
in the linen closet where it remained hidden until its weekly
appearance. To spare me the difficult task, my sweet husband
administered the injections. Saturday night "shot time" became
an unexpected weekly bonding ritual that served as yet another
harsh reminder of our devoted commitment. We alternated
legs and injection sites at the suggestion of the nurse trainer.
Sometimes the shots were virtually pain-free. Other times I
experienced an intense sting. If Scott hit a blood vessel, the
amount of squirting or oozing was matched with his regretful
apology. I knew it wasn't his fault, and I always thanked him
no matter what. My groom was definitely fulfilling his end of the
wedding vows as we hoped for a stable outlook over the next
eight years of injections. Even though no one can see into the
future, I felt confident about taking one step to hopefully control
and prevent future progression.

At this point, I've given up the shots and opted for a
newer oral form of my chosen therapy. No more needles for

me. The only side effect I experienced with this new drug was what the package insert describes as occasional "flushing." It actually feels more like a four alarm fire! Fortunately, it rarely happens now, but occasionally if I take the pill on an empty stomach, I can feel a hot sensation climbing up my body and creeping through my scalp. If Scott or Reece are around when it happens, they'll announce, "She's an Oompa Loompa! Quick, how about some peanut butter or applesauce before you explode into flames!" When I look in the mirror, I have to giggle as I imagine Reece dialing 911 to report his pre-combustion Mom-ergency!

When I transitioned to this oral med, the same friendly nurse explained the gradual adjusted dosing process. Because I was busy and thought I knew it all after years of injections, I didn't pay as much attention to her explanation about the pills as I did for the shot training. They're pills...how hard could they be? I relayed what I remembered about the dosage instructions to Scott who loads my grandma-like pill and vitamin organizer each week. By 10 a.m. every morning, I was turning chili pepper red until we realized Scott was using the wrong bottle and inadvertently DOUBLING my dosage instead of reducing it by half! Through laughter and relief, I jokingly accused him of trying to poison me. Since we figured it out, it's been smooth sailing with only the occasional empty stomach Oompa Loompa appearance. Fortunately between the drug manufacturer and my insurance company, this current DMD, which has a whopping cost of $55,000 per year is now covered at 100%!

As grateful as I am to have access to an effective drug option, I'm still annoyed that millions of research dollars are spent creating new drugs to slow progression and treat symptoms when a cure remains elusive. Occasionally, I wonder if all the MS walks and bike rides will really ever lead to a cure. I also question whether big pharma just wants us to keep popping their pills and injecting their needles in order to continuously and generously line shareholder pockets. However, I waste very little energy with such toxic thoughts which only occur when I'm feeling sorry for myself and cursing MS. Research has come very far just since I was diagnosed. Now with all the DMD options and so much research focused on unraveling the mysteries of this disease, as bizarre as this sounds, there is no better time in history to be diagnosed with MS.

Therefore I remain hopeful that progress will continue, and that within my lifetime, we will be able to prevent and actually cure the disease. It might involve myelin repair or stem cells rather than a drug, but for now, I take a DMD as a sort of insurance policy -- akin to wearing a seatbelt while driving. It's been proven to slow progression, and since taking it, I haven't developed any new lesions which makes me very grateful to my chosen drug manufacturer. So until a better option presents itself, I will continue taking it but won't rely solely on my neurologist or the drug alone. It's my job to take control of my mind and body by ensuring that my suit of armor is strong on all fronts -- not just one.

MS is defined by questions without many answers. After more than two decades with a disease that has attempted to take away my control, I've made the decision to focus on what I *can* control. Just like Jack Canfield's *Success Principles*, I take "100% responsibility" for how well I defend my mind and my body against further progression of MS.

A daily coping mechanism that provides some instant satisfaction is that I cuss colorfully in my mind. Normally no one hears it, but in the midst of a struggle, my silent f-bombs are flying, and the expletives do slightly cushion my ungraceful crashes. When facing adversity, however, I needed better options.

Another habit that has become a refuge is meditation. Until I experienced it for myself, I didn't understand what it entailed or how it might be beneficial. The whole concept was foreign to me, and I thought I was far too busy to make time for something that frivolous. I associated meditation with monks and incense, but what I've discovered is meditation helps to retrain my brain to be still and present. Instead of always spinning my wheels about what's happening tomorrow or what happened yesterday, it keeps me in the here and now and better equipped to process all that's being thrown at me on a daily basis. The mindfulness and calm that meditation creates is also invaluable for my ADD-like tendencies and is much healthier than the alternatives.[2] When I don't have time

---

2   https://news.harvard.edu/gazette/story/2018/04/harvard-researchers-study-how-mindfulness-may-change-the-brain-in-depressed-patients/

for a 15-minute session, I practice the One Breath meditation experience that takes less than one minute and can be done anywhere, anytime, and even with my eyes open so no one even knows.[3] It brings light and reduces anxiety when I'm in traffic or waiting on an infinite hold with my insurance company or cell phone carrier. When I do make the time for some stillness, a meditation app on my phone is always ready. It's a refreshing and powerful way to spend a few moments simply focusing on my breath when I need clarity. While meditation is great, I needed even more tools.

We've all heard that laughter is the best medicine. Fortunately, I had grown up watching my parents propel through their own stumbles with a good dose of laughter. While my mother's natural inclination was to be plagued by worry, it was often tempered by my clever dad's powerful sense of humor. She worried non-stop about everything imaginable. Dad worried about nothing. Her constant state of concern meant a need to hear a detailed weather forecast multiple times a day. She thrived on her awareness of tracking heat waves, cold snaps, storms, and other drastic weather patterns. I received many a phone call over the years warning me of severe weather conditions headed my way. As my husband is also fascinated by weather, between the two of them, I never needed a weather radio. Even though he didn't understand it, my dad was amused by this obsession. Many times I heard him say,

---

3   http://www.wellnesstips.ca/one%20breath%20meditation.htm

"The weather is going to do what the weather is going to do if you worry about it or not, Marion." In her defense, maybe she truly found the meteorological science behind weather to be intriguing. Even so, she wasted mounds of energy fretting about the weather as well as other things she couldn't control.

Like the weather, I can't control my disease, so while meditation has often helped ease my situation, humor almost always provides relief. I rely on it daily, especially when facing the frustrating desire to do more than my body will allow. Fortunately, finding the comedy in sometimes random situations is a skill I developed years ago to move forward with a smile no matter what's happening around me. Sometimes it's uncontrollably spontaneous like the time I chuckled inappropriately at a funeral. Something tickled my funny bone, and my body literally became unable to control the response. I don't remember what caused it, but I doubt it was that funny.

To this day, I have to laugh when I think of another particularly ill-timed case of silliness from many years ago. As newlyweds, Scott and I signed up for a "Marriage Enrichment Seminar." As my interpretation of enrichment is taking something good and making it even better, I wrongly assumed this seminar was intended for couples who wanted to "enrich" an already healthy relationship. Not only is that untrue for "enriched" cereal, but it was definitely not the case for this event. It was a more weighty and intense experience than expected to say the least.

As each couple shared their expectations for the day, it was obvious we had a very different relationship than the other attendees. While we enjoyed blissful newlywed contentedness, most of the couples had been married for many years and seemed to have deeply rooted conflicts. One couple even revealed to the group that this was the last stop in repairing their troubled relationship before divorce. We were instructed to separate into couples and take turns divulging our feelings of hurt or betrayal with our partner. Boxes of tissues were placed around the room in anticipation of tears. I couldn't help but eavesdrop on a couple as they delved into feelings that likely involved an affair. Once we got to this point, we weren't sure how to bow out gracefully. So instead, we followed the directions and desperately tried to uncover something troubling about our relationship to no avail.

About that time, I was distracted by a whistling noise that I presumed was coming from the loudly humming wall air conditioning unit. However, after the air stopped blowing, the whistle continued. Scott saw my look of confusion as I tried to pinpoint the source of the whistle, and eventually I could tell that he heard it now, too. I couldn't concentrate on what we were supposed to be discussing as our eyes darted around the room, searching for the source of the sound. At almost the same moment, our eyes locked as we realized where the sound originated. Every time one of the spouses seated across the room took a breath, his nose loudly whistled. We looked around the room at the other faces obviously engrossed in their conversations and oblivious to the whistle. It was gaining volume and sounded like a teapot boiling on the stove. I attempted to stifle my laughter with a fake coughing fit as I left the room in search of a bathroom where I could release my pent up laughter. It's certainly one of those moments that we will always remember and surely broke the tension of the day.

At my recent bi-annual neuro appointment with Dr. R, we both chuckled at what might sound like dire information to most. I asked her a question that I'd been wondering but had never asked before: How many lesions did I actually have anyway? Her response was, "Too many to count." I replied, "I can count all the way to 100, and I bet with all your schooling you can too." After giggling, she explained that when there are more than 20 plaques, they stop counting. I didn't imagine having an uncountable number but as the literal definition of multiple sclerosis is "multiple scars," what did I expect?

It doesn't really matter if I have 76 or 276 splotches. One thing that does matter is keeping a sense of humor. Lauren, a fellow MSer I met online during the holiday season shared that her MRI films look like a snow globe. That tickled my funny bone as her description painted a vivid and very timely picture. She followed with this, "I'm dreaming of a white Christmas." Ba du bum. Now that's the kind of perspective this craziness requires.

During conversations in the kitchen, my husband has turned around on more than one occasion to find me on the floor. Out of nowhere, the floor seems to just reach up and grab me, and as long as there are no broken bones or blood involved, it can be quite funny. Perhaps not to my husband or anyone else, but it is to me. Trust me, the first time it happened, I wasn't laughing either, but now it happens so frequently that I can almost see myself crumpling to the floor as if I'm observing from afar, and it makes me laugh hysterically. Fortunately, I've become skilled at falling. When you stumble to the ground regularly, like an adventure-flick stuntwoman, your fall expertise improves. I've often said, after practically bouncing back up after a fall, "I do all my own stunts."

Even the sting of embarrassment has, at times, been softened by a little humor. When I used to walk down a hallway pre-walker and someone came toward me, it was my natural tendency to be friendly and look them in the eye with a smile. The problem with that, however, is that my feet tend to go where my eyes do, so I would invariably veer in their direction. I'm like a pinball bouncing off the walls. I started, not so lovingly, referring to these occurrences as gravity pulls. On several occasions I nearly crashed into a confused passerby who must have been unnerved by a surprise attack from the crazy drunk lady. I would apologize and quickly explain that I had "balance issues." After those nearly disastrous close-calls, I would continue down the hallway with a frenzy of confused mental cuss words intertwined with giggles as I recalled the horrified expressions on their faces. After all, they had experienced the trauma of someone flagrantly abusing the rules of unspoken hallway etiquette. I now push my walker which helps eliminate such catastrophes and is evidence that I'm not just inebriated or insane. Even though it's not my nature, I've also learned to forgo friendly eye contact. To maintain my forward trajectory, my focus must remain straight ahead determinedly focused on the destination or it may get ugly.

I have been known to flash a mean stink-eye stare at particularly rude and troublesome flooring that unexpectedly rises up like an ocean wave to knock me off my feet. And the reaction on my face when a cantankerous vertical door frame shoves into me is Oscar worthy! After the initial silent curse word in my brain, I just chuckle at the ridiculousness of this whole thing. While I'm certainly not claiming all the miserable MS symptoms I struggle with are laughable, it has been helpful and reassuring to find the humor in otherwise pitiful situations. Humor didn't always come so easily, especially after I was newly diagnosed and later when I was first feeling the deterioration of my body. Since becoming a reluctant expert on navigating hardship, I've realized the undeniable therapy of laughter. I empathetically understand why many of our greatest comedians came from a background of struggle. Wouldn't we all rather laugh than cry? I read an autobiography written by one of my favorite funny ladies, Carol Burnett, whose sketch comedy antics made me roar with laughter as a kid. She's quoted as insightfully saying, "Comedy = Tragedy + Time."

When you really break it down, we're all pretty hilarious beings. The things we so often get tied up in knots about are usually temporary and probably won't matter to us or anyone else when on our deathbeds. I often use this "impending death" litmus test to remind myself of what's truly important so that I remain in the driver's seat. When I'm at the very end, will it matter that I ran into the door frame, fell down and skinned my knee or wet my pants? Nine out of ten times the answer is no, and that is an incredibly valuable perspective.

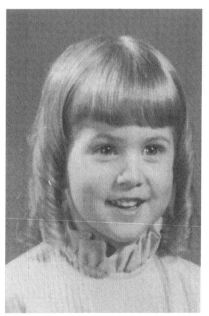
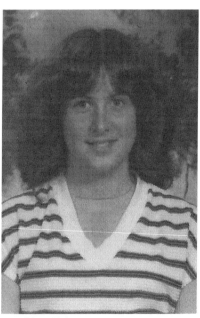

Me with Tish   *Me without Tish*

CHAPTER SEVEN

Recalculating

You can believe the diagnosis, not the prognosis.

~ Deepak Chopra

Symptom management has become the gold standard of efficacy for almost every drug on the market. With a perplexing condition like MS, most of the medicines I've taken through the years aren't treating my disease, they're helping to relieve a symptom. If it's pain, insomnia, fatigue, depression, incontinence, worsening gait, tremors, etc. a neurologist will be happy to write a prescription. When I've been given free samples in my doc's office, I felt as lucky as if I hit the lottery -- wow, FREE drugs! The trouble I encountered with many of these pills is that the side effects were sometimes as bad as the problem they were supposed to address and merely attempted to mask what was happening in my body. It's worth tolerating a side effect or two if the original problem was at least addressed. Many times, that wasn't the case. Frustratingly, the side effects appeared, but the symptom didn't improve.

Trust me, I appreciate relief when it's needed but what about improving me? I'm the person behind the frustrating symptom. My doctor only sees the outward signs of my MS. It's up to me to improve what's going on inside. I don't blindly accept that our own FDA has tested and approved the only possible treatment options for all conditions. With any affliction, my first inclination is to find alternative therapies for whatever is happening to me or someone I love. As I look in new directions, I'm amazed at what I learn about spiritual healing through the power of the mind-body connection. I believe there is useful wisdom in the thousands of years of experience of ancient ayurvedic and traditional Chinese medicine and have experienced relief and benefits from non-traditional treatments like acupuncture, massage, CBD oil and essential oils to name a few. These treatments help put my mind and body in a happy place, and even if some of the benefits are only short lived, any type of prevention and therapy is a highly valued gift. Organic coconut oil and apple cider vinegar are just two of my favorite go-to healing substances that are inexpensive and have been treating and preventing ailments for centuries. Just as I am more than my disease, I must remain a vigilant and open-minded health student, always learning so that I put up a good fight against the MonSter while becoming the healthiest version of me that I can be.

We are a combination of what we eat, how we move, and how we think. Besides my outlook, what's made the biggest and most consistent impact on the way I feel has nothing to do with pills, oils, or needles. It's the simple brilliance of clean eating and daily exercise.

We hear the echoing choruses touting various diet and exercise plans from TV and internet personalities ad nauseum. Each one professes their strategy is the best. I question how they know what my body needs compared to the next person they meet who has a completely different set of circumstances. How do they know what it feels like to be me? Do they truly understand that just taking a shower, making the bed, or making dinner are frequently dreaded, overwhelming tasks? On those difficult days when my body seems extra MonSter-ish, the idea of "laying like broccoli" as Julia Roberts says in *Pretty Woman* is tempting. Staying in my comfy chair and playing the MS card crosses my mind, but when I stand up and let my spastic, unsure legs stretch and begin to move, I realize I always feel better when I'm done exercising. It may seem counterintuitive with my limited energy, but a consistent dose of simple physical activity keeps me feeling like a fighter instead of a victim.

I learned the importance of exercise from my dad who

ran two miles every other day for as long as I can remember. He jogged at a slow and steady pace in rain, snow, ice, and heat. The weather didn't stop him. In fact, nothing did until he was 84 and Alzheimer's meant he couldn't remember his way home from the old road behind our house. When I bragged on him through the years, he humbly professed that he wasn't doing anything remarkable. I thought differently. I certainly didn't know anyone whose father jogged every other day at the age of 50, 60, 70, and especially at 80! Through his example, I learned the value of consistent exercise: when you keep your body moving, it can be stronger and more defensive. Even though he couldn't defend his mind against the eventual ravages of dementia, he was able to enjoy his highly active life until Alzheimer's really took hold. It's notable, too, that until then, he also never required the plethora of prescription drugs often found on the kitchen counters of most older Americans.

As for my dad-inspired workouts, they've definitely changed over time. Admittedly, I spent a few years post diagnosis in denial but not in complacency. I learned from my father and took action not by just joining a gym but showing up there almost daily which is half the battle. Like Dad, I was consistent, but that doesn't mean I was skilled. I'll never forget when a trainer at my old fitness center pulled me into a gym to join his boot camp class that was starting in 10 minutes. Apparently he saw me there often and wanted me to experience one of his classes in hopes that I might become a regular. I resisted and told him I didn't know if I could keep up because I had MS. Either he had no idea what I was talking about or thought I said PMS because he responded nonchalantly, "No big deal. And don't worry, I'm not going to charge you for this class." He didn't give me much of a choice as he pulled my arm while I played along to avoid appearing wimpy. It was, after all, free! The other five women in the class seemed to be at varying fitness levels, so I thought I might be able to fit in somewhere.

I was wrong. I struggled through the high intensity workout even though my body couldn't make quick moves like the others. I'm the girl who has to concentrate on just walking, so my brain definitely couldn't keep up with the rapid-fire movements through the peanut butter and ocean waves! When he wasn't looking, I opted for shortcuts and took rests instead of repetitions. With nothing for support and trying to ignore my uncooperative body, I fell several times while lunging from one end of the gym to the other. I'm still not sure how I survived that class without broken bones, but it reinforced that exercise is an individual endeavor. Just because someone else my age can do it doesn't mean I can. I was a gym member for many years, but in time, my legs would become exhausted from just preparing, driving there, and getting into the big facility. My workout was over before it ever began.

My alternative these days is having basic exercise equipment at home which also means no extra time, money, or energy is wasted getting to my destination or paying for a membership. The best part is I don't have to worry about how I look among the sea of protein-obsessed fitness buffs. I simply lace up my sneakers and can be on my stationary bike or elliptical in minutes. I rotate days from upper or lower body weight-resistance exercises. Maintaining strength is obviously important for all of us as we age, but I have an additional reason to fight muscle loss.

During my exercises, every move I make must be supported. No more walking lunges or free-standing dead lifts like I used to do. While making the necessary accommodations to each move is simple, it does require some planning and, at times, even instruction from a pro. I also pace myself by doing smaller sessions rather than pushing my limits like I used to do at the gym. If I'm shooting for 20 minutes of cardio, it doesn't matter to me if 10 minutes happen in the morning and the other 10 in the afternoon. Every day for me is different so I just listen to what my body tells me it can handle. Some days I feel invincible and am astounded by what I can do, but most days I barely struggle through.

I have to admit I despise exercise. I'm only able to make these workouts happen because of my desire to get each one behind me. When they're over, I'm in heaven. After each workout session, my legs usually feel like mush as I fall to the ground celebrating that I'm done. My greatest satisfaction is getting back on my feet and hitting my big red "Easy" button that announces in a deep voice, "That was easy." I suppose that's my way of thumbing my nose at MS and saying, "I am not lying down and letting you have your way with me! I'll show you who's boss!" I relish the satisfaction it gives me, and I end up feeling empowered and confident even on less than ideal days.

Because I'm not certified in personal training, I've benefited from following along with various YouTube videos for direction. When I need more structure and guidance, I've periodically hired trainers to come to my home or visited PT's to help lay out specific exercise plans that will work for me. As they teach me the moves, I ask them to write down an explanation of that activity on an index card using words that will make sense to me later. Otherwise, I would surely enter my workout room the next day and completely blank out on what I was supposed to be doing, especially if they use a technical term to refer to an exercise. A hip abduction? Someone is trying to steal my hip? Instead, I prefer them to spell out that I need to lay on my side with legs stretched out straight, then raise and hold the top leg for five counts for two sets of 20. Without clear instructions, I could never remember a single thing they showed me. Instead, I pick up that day's card and confidently get down to business while already looking forward to my Easy button, of course. With the online resources these days, options abound. It's just a matter of a few keystrokes to find different workouts when I need a change.

Every session begins and ends with deep breathing and stretching, and it feels so good. Learning how to breathe is powerful and who would imagine that our bodies could be trained to breathe correctly? Deep controlled breathing, followed by stretching, gets my blood flowing and helps my stiff body move a little better throughout the day. I have enough physical challenges without being tight and cramped. After a cardio warm up, I always incorporate leg stretches, a cobra stretch, and planking. Maintaining core strength is a necessity for everyone, but especially for someone with balance issues. I'm now dabbling in yoga and look forward to expanding more in that direction. As always, I remain an open-minded, lifelong learner and plan to continue investigating different types of workouts, ideas, and equipment. When we think we know it all, we can become stuck and not able to move past our current situation. It goes a step further for me. Once I stop moving, I have a fear of eternally being stuck in one place. I continue learning and moving my body in order to sustain my mobility and independence which are both valiant motivators.

With or without MS, we are all at different fitness and ability levels. While my current workouts might seem very remedial and unchallenging for a true fitness buff, I don't claim to be a competitive weightlifter or olympian. When doing something to move, stretch, and lift, even while sitting, the reward is that I will feel better mentally and physically.

Once I lost the ability to walk long distances or balance on a bicycle, my exercise was limited to the indoor variety. On a trail ride several years ago, I lost my balance and crashed to the pavement, skinning my knees and elbows in a scene reminiscent of a four-year-old whose training wheels were just removed. After that, I was done. No more cycling for me. Walking had become hazardous enough; I certainly didn't need to add an additional source of injury to my life. Ironically, biking is my husband's favorite hobby so for my birthday last year, he surprised me with a new TRICYCLE! I could ride yet feel balanced and stable with no risk of falling thanks to those three wheels. Feeling the fresh air and independence was overwhelming and brought tears to my eyes as I pedaled down the street. I could care less how geeky I look. I'm closer to 50 than 5 and love my trike!

I've benefited not only by the power of consistent exercise but by learning how to hold my body correctly. When I mentioned to Kelly, my knowledgeable trainer, that standing worsened my pain, she immediately observed my lousy posture and showed me the proper stance required to relieve pressure on the back. She said to visualize a rope running up parallel with my spine and being pulled straight above my head and to pretend that my two rib cages were interlocking like the fingers of both hands clasping and intertwining together. Then she said to hold my core tight as if I was expecting to be punched in the gut. It's such a simple idea, but I'm continually amazed how much this small adjustment has impacted my life. When I "forget" my posture rules, I can feel it. We are, after all, highly complex machines made up of many functioning parts that periodically need realignment to operate smoothly.

The bottom line is that exercise, just like food and water, are critical for our bodies. Like my dad, I know that my workouts might not be remarkable, and even though I don't look forward to them, I do them anyway. That "Easy" button feels spectacular because of what it represents! I may not win any competitions, but I am taking control of what I can control to live the best life possible..

Even though I didn't choose this disease, I do have a daily choice before me.

- I can succumb to the difficulties I face and become a victim.

OR

- I can choose NOT to allow MS to have the power. I will lead my life, thank you.

That's my job -- not MS's!

CHAPTER EIGHT

Keeping It Simple

The doctor of the future will give no medicine, but will interest his patients in the care of the human body, in diet, and in the cause and prevention of disease.

~ Thomas Edison

Those who experience constant chronic pain know it becomes crippling and life-altering. A few years ago, I was ravaged by unrelenting neurologic pain that is sometimes referred to as the "MS Hug." A better name would be the MS Torture Crush. Hugs are nice, but this hug is not. It felt like a vice squeezing my upper body while a sharp knife stabbed at me and hot flames shot from my back. Even breathing hurt. When the miserable sensation first began, I thought my bra was too tight. I went from a 34 to 36 to 38 band size searching for relief, but the bigger sizes did not change the way I felt. By noon each day, the pain level was off the charts. This lasted for many years and impacted my personality.

Because of my very social profession, I often had to draw upon my acting skills to function successfully. Even though I was crying inside with pain, I continued to smile and work like nothing was pressing upon me. My poor husband Scott, however, is the one who saw the real, miserable me. When I came home from a work event, I would collapse, sometimes in tears, from the pain and fatigue. We often let our guard down around those we love the most, and for a few years, I wasn't the fun, joyful person he had married.

I couldn't sleep and became addicted to my nightly dose of Ambien to knock me out. Lack of sleep, of course, makes everything worse, so I welcomed the drug-induced, pain-free nights. The puzzle of neurological pain is difficult for doctors to treat (or solve), and I was prescribed various drugs as they guessed which one might work. None of them did. As my drug options dwindled, my neurologist tried using meds that were originally developed for other various conditions, but nothing brought relief. I kept popping the pills anyway because I saw no other option. To make it worse, a few of them caused horrible side effects. I was in a bad cycle and didn't see a way out.

When I was at the worst of this physically wretched time, I had a conversation with Scott. I told him that if this misery was going to be my new normal for the rest of my life, I didn't have the desire to be on this earth long-term. I couldn't take another 20 or 30 years of this, so once I saw our son graduate college, I would be ready to call it quits. The constant pain changed who I was and stole my typically sunny outlook.

When you're already down and out, things invariably get worse before they get better. I was attending a business meeting at my company's North American headquarters near Boston when I contracted pneumonia. I felt awful as I delivered a live-feed video presentation being viewed by the top leaders in my company. My thespian skills helped me struggle through the 20 minute speech and what should have been an enjoyable and delicious seafood dinner afterward. Later, alone in a hotel room, I knew something was horribly wrong but I wasn't thinking straight. I was freezing and nearly delirious lying in bed when I realized I had to pee. I tried to stand up but rolled to the floor instead. My legs would not work, so I crawled on all fours to the bathroom and pushed myself up on the side of the toilet. When I was done, I frantically crawled back to the bed. Though my legs still weren't functioning the next morning, I had to pack and catch a plane. I called to the front desk and told them I was having a medical problem and needed a wheelchair and their help with packing. No, I didn't want them to call 911, I just needed some help so I could get home to my own bed. I was out of it with a high fever and don't remember all the details. What I do remember is Susan, a kind business comrade, looking at me in shock as the hotel staff transported me through the lobby and out to a waiting cab. She accompanied me as I slept all the way to the airport and then helped me check in for my miserable flight. I couldn't think of anything other than getting to my bed. Somehow I retrieved my car in the extended parking lot but not without backing up and crumpling my rear bumper into a concrete divider before paying my parking fee. As I drove on the interstate and to my house, I was barely able to focus on the road. I remember hoping that I wouldn't run into the median or endanger the other drivers. I went through the motions to get home to my sacred bed where I remained and battled the vicious illness for six long weeks.

Scott immediately came home and started treating my 105 degree temperature. When you have MS and you experience extreme heat or cold, every one of your worst MS related symptoms may intensify to a new level. Entire body systems can be affected or even shut down. In my case, when my body temp rises even one degree, my legs decide to take a hiatus. With ongoing extremely high fevers, I could barely walk and the pain from my MS hug was excruciating. While lying in bed, I heard television news reports about the intensity of that year's pneumonia epidemic leading to multiple deaths across the country. I imagined the relief that the end would bring and asked Scott if he was aware of my preferred funeral arrangements. The poor guy was single-handedly taking care of me and our then six-year-old son while also running our household and still working his full-time job. He didn't want to hear it. He could see beyond the pneumonia even when I couldn't. One of the only things that helped me survive that time were the nightly St Louis Cardinal games. We were on a winning streak and made it to the World Series, eventually coming out as the national champs! Their games along with the love of my two favorite guys provided a much needed distraction from my agony.

I survived pneumonia, but the pattern of relentless pain and rounds of various ineffective prescriptions continued. A few years later, my oldest sister, Becca, called me one July day with some interesting news. She'd been on vacation and read a book about the benefits of eliminating gluten and eating clean. I'd heard the term "gluten free" before but had no idea what it meant. She said she was giving it a try as she suffered from rheumatoid arthritis (RA), another autoimmune condition, and wondered if this modification could have a positive impact on her health. The RA was wreaking havoc on her joints and her ability to function each day.

I wished her well and told her to keep me posted but doubted her wild idea would work. Besides, MS had taken much from me, and I wasn't going to let food be another stolen pleasure. I enjoyed bread, cookies, pasta, cereal, and cake and wasn't willing to part ways with any of them. I mindlessly snacked on candy throughout the day and every evening I enjoyed a big bowl of ice cream that was usually accompanied by chocolate sauce or brownies. I justified it by purchasing low-fat ice cream and believing that my consistent dose of daily exercise counteracted my sweet-toothed obsession. I felt horrible, but my dependency was at least giving me a small measure of joy though not providing me anything approaching real comfort or relief.

When my sister reported back that her joint functioning was improving and she felt better overall, I reluctantly agreed to take a closer look. After all, genetically speaking, she was the closest possible DNA profile match to mine. If it was positively impacting my own sister who, like me, had an autoimmune disease, then I owed it to myself to investigate.

I did the research and concluded I had to go for it. I learned about many others with various autoimmune conditions who were also benefitting from a radical food shift. I studied functional medicine doctors who explained that fueling our bodies with refined grains and added sugars was contributing to the inflammation and declining health of Americans. I was devastated, however, about giving up the foods I loved. Once again, I asked my wise son who was eight years old at the time for his input. I told him that Aunt Becca was feeling much better since she changed her diet and explained that if I tried the same thing, I would need to give up all of my favorites like bread, cookies, and cake. I'll never forget his response: "Mom, you've had cake before, but you haven't been pain-free in a long time." My young son's straightforward response influenced my decision. He was right, and I kept repeating his words of wisdom. I'd eaten plenty of cake in my life, but the idea of possibly improving the way I felt sounded more delicious than any dessert I had ever tasted.

Since I was being bulldozed by a medical crisis, it was time to take control and play offense. The most obvious place for me to take charge was by analyzing what I put in my mouth. Much research is proving that inflammation causes the demyelination of the nerves in people with MS and that certain foods cause inflammation.[4] Therefore, why not avoid those foods and add the ones that reduce it? With all this in mind, I jumped in with hopeful gusto. I got rid of all the highly processed garbage food in our house by donating it, giving it to neighbors or throwing it away. I was on a mission. Even though ingredients are clearly listed on food packages, I didn't take time to read them all. If the ingredients list was long and if I couldn't pronounce the 15-letter words, I tossed it. I made a plan that included only simple, clean foods free of gluten, refined sugar, and dairy, plus loads of vegetables and high-quality fats. This wasn't something I could do halfway. I knew that if I truly wanted to determine the results of my experiment, I would need to be entirely committed. It was all or nothing, so I made no excuses. If I was going out to eat or to a social gathering, I would eat an avocado, vegetables, and nuts beforehand so I'd eliminate hunger and make smart choices.

4   https://www.mindbodygreen.com/articles/the-top-foods-that-cause-inflammation

There were some physical challenges, the first of which was the sugar withdrawal. I've since learned that for some people, sugar can be as addictive as cocaine. I certainly thought it was during that first couple of weeks when I felt tortuously deprived. Just like a smoker who goes cold turkey, the cravings were intense. Because sugar is a "natural" and "low-fat" substance, I always assumed it was safe. Heck, I even grew up singing the "C&H Pure Cane Sugar, from Hawaii, grown in the sun" song. The more I read, however, the more I suspected that sugar was toxic to me and probably many others. Some research I read even went so far as to claim cancer, obesity, Alzheimer's, diabetes, heart disease, and autoimmune conditions all have links to sugar. (See *The Case Against Sugar* by Gary Taubes.) It's often added in one of its various forms to nearly every box, bag, and jar we choose from the middle of the supermarket. Of course, when we're hooked, we buy more. Could food manufacturers be preying on our sweet-toothed obsessions? I didn't have time to wait for the results of unlikely lifelong, double blind studies to find out how our bodies will be impacted by lifetimes of poor choices. I took action.

With any goal, I knew that a measurable time frame was vital. One month was my initial benchmark, but just after a few weeks, I saw positive results. My pain was significantly reduced, so I committed to another month of clean eating. By that time, I was over the sugar hump and decided to go for a full year! Once I had completed a year of this new lifestyle, I would celebrate.

Miraculously, after a year of whole, simple foods without processed sugar, my pain was virtually gone, and I was amazed. No longer was I trapped in that painful existence. I was in control of my health — not food or MS! I could focus on fun, family, and work without misery even entering the picture. Occasionally, I would just stop in total disbelief and really observe how I felt. Every day by noon, my pain level used to be a 10 on a scale of one to 10, but after my food shift, I only noticed the pain when I looked for it. I might be up to a pain level of two or three later in the day after too much standing or exposure to high heat or stress, but on a normal day, I was pain free. I was a believer! While I might forever be a member of Sugars Anonymous, the benefits of my new life greatly exceed that of my old miserable days eating highly processed, sugar-laden "food-like" substances.

Interestingly, my taste buds adjusted accordingly and my sugar cravings evaporated. After several years, I do, on a special occasion, sample a now off-limits dessert or snack. I refuse to miss out on birthday parties or holiday fun which most often revolve around food. When I do, though, I find that even birthday cake is not as appealing as it used to be. My taste for these foods has nearly disappeared since I know what they contain. In fact, at times I've quietly spit offending food into my napkin. I know that's gross, but I now think highly enough of myself that I have no desire to ingest such low quality, pain and inflammation-causing junk.

The positive impacts of my new food strategy continued. I dropped pain medications and learned in the process how scary these drugs are. Weaning myself from neurological pain pills was a monumental task. I experienced frightening electric shockwaves in my brain as I gradually cut back the dosage to eventually be pain-med free. It was a daunting process but well worth it. I also fought through and conquered my 14-year sleeping pill habit and found that I actually slept better and longer when I wasn't dependent on the artificial sedative effect of sleeping pills. Busting out of that painful prison has been liberating! When I reported these results to my doctors and canceled all pain and sleeping pill prescriptions, they looked at me with serious skepticism. According to a report by the American Medical Association, only 27% of US medical schools actually offer students the recommended 25 hours of nutritional training, so in my doctor's defense, their expertise is NOT nutrition.[5] While I value and appreciate MDs for their knowledge and skill, I don't give them blind authority. My unique body is the only one I've got, so it's up to me to take the lead by educating and advocating for myself to improve my health and my life. New scientific studies support the results of my experience, proving that MS, like many chronic illnesses, can be affected by careful management of diet and exercise.[6]

5   https://wire.ama-assn.org/education/whats-stake-nutrition-education-during-med-school

6   https://www.nationalmssociety.org/Research/Research-News-Progress/Research-News/ECTRIMS2018

It's curious that people will invest so much time and money into purchasing the best possible car on the market. Then they spend even more money to ensure their investment has the best maintenance and care possible. Meanwhile, these same discerning consumers might claim that eating healthy is too expensive, treating their own bodies like garage sale leftovers by filling up on low-quality lab-created foods. Regrettably, the price of leaving themselves vulnerable to breakdown and disease is far greater. It is a fascinating irony that we offer better care to our possessions than ourselves.

It's been said that our genes load the gun but our choices pull the trigger. As a result, I now live by a set of guidelines that I call "Eight is Great." I don't claim to have all the answers for anyone else but this list has definitely helped me clearly define my new lifestyle:

1. If the list of ingredients is long or full of unpronounceable words, get rid of it.

2. Organic leafy greens and colorful vegetables should be the majority of every meal and snack opportunity -- breakfast included.

3. Include healthy fat at every meal and snack. My daily go-to choices are eggs, nuts, seeds, avocados, legumes, good quality olive, coconut and avocado oils, plus occasional grass-fed beef and wild-caught salmon. Other meat should be small servings, high quality, and minimally

processed.

4. Eliminate refined sugar and artificial sweeteners and, when needed, replace with a touch of date, coconut sugar, raw honey or pure maple syrup.

5. Limit dairy to a small amount of good quality cheese or Greek yogurt once or twice a week.

6. Eat grains sparingly and live a gluten-free life with real food and not "gluten free" labeled food. If it has a label that says gluten free, it's probably highly processed.

7. Avoid quasi-food that is cheap, fast, and served through windows. My family and I are worth spending a few more dollars on for real food.

8. Eat berries daily; all other fruits, seasonally and in moderation.

Most importantly, I never think of this as a diet. I don't focus on what I've eliminated but instead concentrate on the abundance of high quality food I've added. Just like my label aversion, my food relationship doesn't fit into any current fad diet plan. I just eat mindfully and enjoy real food and the great purpose it serves. The point of this list is to keep it simple. It's what I believe food should be based on and what I've discovered works for me. When I have doubts, I refer back to my list. With my "Eight is Great," I'm never hungry. I'm not eating less but better, and of course, losing weight was a positive side effect.

Eliminating the inflammation-producing stuff I once craved also meant that I felt more energetic, my digestion was better, and my skin never looked so clear and smooth. For years, my vanity inspired me to spend loads of money on multi-step, pricey topical skin care regimens, but nothing ever made much difference. Blotchiness, adult acne, and uneven skin tone all magically disappeared when I remedied it from the inside. I wasn't searching for those positive "side effects," but they were welcome results of my new lifestyle. According to Stastista, by 2024 the global skin care market is expected to be $180 billion.[7] I once contributed to those statistics when I searched for perfect skin care products. Likewise, weight loss companies who create fortunes marketing their special pre-portioned frozen meals or scientifically created shakes and bars are merely taking advantage of people's aversion to clean, fresh, simple eating. It's not their fault for selling; it's our fault for buying.

In today's medical world, when things go wrong, most of us search for a pill that we naively hope will fix the problem. I sure did, but what I found is that most prescription and over-the-counter drugs came with hefty side effects and only occasional relief. The pills didn't treat me as a whole person. They merely put a Band-Aid on a symptom. I often tell people I'm the healthiest sick person they'll ever meet. I still have MS and don't claim that the lesions covering my brain and spinal cord have disappeared. I still take my DMD faithfully, but I'm

---

7   https://www.statista.com/statistics/254612/global-skin-care-market-size/

confident that choosing high quality sustenance has provided an extra layer of defense against any additional inflammatory attacks on my body. This change definitely gave me control over *something* that impacts my future, and I continue to learn. I read, experiment, implement, stumble, and rise as the process continually repeats. I haven't arrived at a certain destination but instead am on a lifelong journey. I don't know all the answers, but I know how to ask good questions. I'm open-minded and willing to listen to new ideas.

While my husband and son have definitely benefited from my newfound relationship with food, they haven't completely transformed their food habits. Before the shift, Scott was plagued by intestinal misery. He visited numerous GI doctors looking for an answer to his Irritable Bowel Syndrome-like symptoms, but they couldn't find an explanation for his troubles. After witnessing my inspiring results and also embracing the gluten and dairy-free lifestyle, he saw a pretty remarkable outcome. I'm sure my very private husband would prefer I not discuss his digestive issues in public, but I can report that even when he occasionally indulges in his old food habits, his body seems to handle it well in small doses. It's when he goes dairy or gluten-overboard that he struggles.

Initially, when my son saw the transformation his mom was undergoing, he joined the junk food boycott. However, that was four years ago, and he's already back to his old, sugar-frosted cereal and carb-craving little self. I refuse to be the parent who forces or completely restricts something that would most likely be rebelled against anyway. I don't require him to eat exactly the way I do and still buy him some of his favorites. Fortunately, he's an unbelievably active child who prefers to run and play outside over video games any day. In spite of his warp-speed metabolism which processes sugar and carbs faster than most of us, I still cringe when he insists on eating garbage. I know it's not ideal for his growing body. In the meantime, I'm at least comforted that he eats lots of veggies and good quality fats as a result of his Momma's well planned whole-food based meals. My hope is that since he's been exposed to a better way, he will make solid choices about his health on his own terms as he gets older.

I thank my sister for showing me how to take control and arm my body against this perplexing autoimmune MonSter that resides in me. When MS was in the driver's seat, I felt like a victim. Misery and hopelessness fueled by a fear of the unknown robbed me of contentment and stole my lightheartedness. I often felt like a bystander in my own life. Now that I am back behind the wheel and steering my body and my mind in the right direction, I feel gloriously in control. By taking complete responsibility of a powerful aspect of my life, I felt empowered, strong, and positive -- like a fighter instead of the punching bag! We have a choice when it comes to the food we eat, and I decided to choose wisely.

CHAPTER NINE

Pre MS -- Building My Suit of Armor

Sometimes you will never know the value of a moment until it
becomes a memory. ~ Dr. Seuss

For anyone who is dealt life altering circumstances, we likely divide our lives into two distinct timeframes -- before and after. For me, it's Pre-MS and Post-MS. Pre-MS defines the easy-going days when -- like trusted soldiers -- my body obediently followed commands without a trace of pain or insubordination. Before the MS mutiny, I was the General. When I meet someone new, they might assume I've always had MS, but this disease is not the whole story, and I am not solely defined by it. I had a life before MS, and

I'm thankful that I have created a full and rewarding life in spite of it. I firmly believe that my experiences before diagnosis prepared me for the harrowing revolt my body has suffered. My pre-MS experiences not only provided me with the mindset to handle it, but as this disease can feel lonely at times, I've had the reinforcement of a caring team around me. I can't imagine going through the shock and ensuing challenges of this journey without my soulmate, family, and friends around me. From birth, I was unwittingly building an army that would someday sustain me throughout my MS battle. Those early years were full of love, fun, activity, and possibilities. My parents instilled in me the self confidence that only unconditional love develops.

The small Southern Illinois town my family called home was a wonderful place to get started. I grew up on 25 sprawling acres which provided plenty of room for the many toys that my dad enjoyed acquiring for his family, and we learned by watching him work and play. He was a one-of-a-kind, joyful, and huge-hearted fellow who marched to the beat of his own drum and never concerned himself with fitting into a mold. He was a humble and inspiring man, and I am truly proud to be his daughter. My father told me daily how much he loved me. (Note: I credit the bond of a father-daughter relationship as the biggest determining factor to the outcome of a woman's self-esteem and interaction with the opposite sex, but that's another book.)

My parents were an impressive team who ran flourishing

businesses together through the years. As much as they loved us kids, we knew their love for one another was the bedrock relationship in the house. Their love story came to life as they courted via the US Mail, penning letters back and forth during my dad's year-and-a-half-long tour of duty in Japan in the early 1950's. (That love story is certainly another book as well.)

She might have rolled her eyes at times, but I don't recall Mom ever objecting to my dad's latest, sometimes bizarre, and usually spontaneous whim about fun or business. He was a master of both. He ran two miles every other day and enjoyed mowing 12 of those 25 acres with his blue timeworn tractor. He had a professionally-equipped woodshop building, vegetable gardens, and gooseberry bushes. In addition to the trampoline, three-wheelers, pogo sticks, stilts, BB guns, ping pong tables, pinball machines, badminton and volleyball sets, and yo-yo's everywhere, dad had tennis and basketball courts as well as a giant steel playground-style jungle gym installed on our property. All of this made for an idyllic and amusing childhood experience.

Dad also operated multiple businesses, several of which were located right on that family acreage. My parents were successful entrepreneurs who developed a solid reputation as fair, honest business people. Consequently, their businesses thrived. There were various buildings on our property, mostly for the extremely successful flooring stores. But through the years, other thriving operations were added as well. These included forklift refurbishing and sales, wood fabrication and sales, antique car restoration, real estate development, and used office furniture sales, just to name a few. My dad specifically chose this plot of land outside city limits so he could run all these disjointed endeavors without interference from city government.

As a result of all this, my parents' business activities were woven into our daily lives. There was always activity at our house with the phone ringing, customers stopping by, and my parents closing deals. With older sisters and a brother, the phone was ringing some more, music and various instruments were playing, and books, science experiments, and homework were everywhere. Laughter and conversation were nonstop. Additionally, there were always friends and dates stopping by, and we seemed to have a revolving door of unexpected visitors. In the days before cell phones and text messages, friends of the family, relatives, or even my parents' business clients would regularly drop in unannounced. No matter what was happening, my mother would welcome them and usually offer them something homemade and delicious while they joined whatever activity or conversation was in progress. This constant liveliness was the backdrop of a unique childhood that I thoroughly enjoyed.

In the summer of 1974, my family's utopian existence was shaken. My sisters and I were happily enjoying one of those long summer days that seem to last forever as a kid. Oh, the sweetness of playing outside long after dusk when the air finally cools and the first day of school is a thousand years in the future. On one particular hot day in July, my 19-year-old brother went boating. My sisters and I were playing in the rocks by the patio when we saw a police car slowly roll up our long driveway. We wondered why the uniformed officer walked right past us to knock on the door. I'll never forget the guttural scream that emerged from my mom's crumpled body or the tears streaming down my usually strong father's heartbroken face. My parents were shaken to the core by the drowning death of their loving, oldest child and only son. Their hearts were torn in pieces that day, and for the rest of their lives, that grief was always present, albeit under the surface and tempered with the passage of time.

My parents still had three daughters and multiple ventures to juggle, so they mourned as they continued with their daily demands. In fact, the commotion of their lives probably aided their ability to function and move forward. After weathering life's most horrific storm, the members of my family didn't sweat the small stuff. If you lost the keys, burned a meal, or wrecked the car, it was not a big deal. When someone did Dad wrong, he didn't get upset. Once when a highly-trusted employee was caught stealing, Dad promptly bailed the guy out of jail, told him he didn't realize he wasn't paying him enough, and actually gave him a raise. He had compassion for those in desperate situations. Coincidentally, the guy never pilfered again.

My parents held us even closer as they had been savagely reminded of the fragility of life. Their love intensified for us girls but also for everyone around them who was doing their best to navigate through life's peaks and valleys. After watching them deal with the greatest tragedy, it was clear that as long as you're living and breathing, virtually nothing is insurmountable. I don't remember us girls whining about much, but if we did, there was very little sympathy given. I've seen kids have meltdowns if the crust of their sandwich barely touched the apples on their lunch plate. When I complained about something inconsequential, my dad would cup his hand under my eyes and with a wry smile would say in a silly voice, "Cry in Daddy's little hand." As infuriating as that was to a hormonal preteen girl, it was clear that whining wouldn't be acknowledged. My family didn't accept any other option than to deal head on with our challenges. I'm certain that my early childhood experience prepared me for the rest of my life.

After high school, I chose a college that was four hours from home so that I could be just far enough away to feel independent while still close enough to commute home in a day. I wasn't attending with a friend from home or rooming with anyone I knew. The college experience was going to be *my* adventure.

The balmy August day that I moved from my childhood home to my freshman dorm was full of kinetic energy and emotion. After my parents helped me lug my belongings into my room, they stayed for a couple of hours. Then we said our tearful goodbyes, and I was on my own. (Disclaimer: As my parents were footing the bill for my entire college expense, I know that doesn't qualify as truly being "on my own." However, that was the first time I had lived under a different roof and in a separate zip code than my parents.)

After a few hours of unpacking and organizing my tiny room, it suddenly hit me that I didn't know a single person on that entire campus. As someone who identifies as a "people person," that was an uncomfortable feeling for me. When I eventually ventured out of my room, I quickly made friends with another freshman in the same situation named Tracy. We paired up and headed to the student center for a slice of pizza -- the sustenance of college students everywhere.

While sitting there and getting to know my new friend in the food court, I noticed a guy I had met at a college preview weekend a few months earlier named Scott. As he was quite good looking, he was hard to forget. I had been introduced to Scott by Darcy, my roommate for the preview weekend. They were both from the same town about an hour away and Darcy was quite giddy when Scott approached us as the preview events got under way. "Oh my gosh! Here he comes. This guy is from my town, and I really like him," she blurted out. Just then

I noticed a tall, dark, and handsome guy walking toward us. As he sauntered up, he gave her a friendly hello. I stood there awkwardly as the two of them exchanged pleasantries, probably both relieved to see a familiar face from home. After a few uncomfortable minutes and as almost an afterthought, Darcy finally said, "Oh Scott, this is my roommate this weekend, Gina."

Just then a university representative quieted the chit chat and announced that all attendees would be divided into small groups based on our declared majors. Scott and I were herded in one direction while Darcy left with a different group. Since we now "knew" each other, we stuck together.

Scott and I chatted throughout the day, and I might have flirted and batted my eyes at him just a little. (He would later admit that my propensity to touch his leg or arm while I was talking piqued his interest in me even more). He had a great smile, warm brown eyes, and manly, muscular legs. He was a good listener and even though he seemed rather quiet, I could see exactly why Darcy liked him. In a lifetime there are a handful of souls that you meet and with whom you immediately feel a connection. With Scott, I felt it.

As he had a younger brother at home who couldn't be left unattended, Scott and his Mom had driven over just for the day and weren't spending the night like most of the incoming freshmen. At the end of the day, we said goodbye, and I went back to my dorm for the night to catch up with Darcy about our big day on campus. I might have skimmed over how much I enjoyed Scott's company.

When he showed up for the next day's preview events, I was happy to see him. His mom had to work so he drove himself which seemed especially grown up to me at the time. After impatiently tolerating endless tours and lectures about what might happen on campus if we weren't completely prepared, we were eventually released for lunch. Scott invited me to join him for a quick meal off campus, and I, of course, didn't hesitate to accept the offer. The conversation was easy, and we both enjoyed being away from the crowd.

We finished up the day by visiting individual stations and signing up for our first semester classes. We were separated in the chaos. After our schedules were printed, we were directed to leave and come back for the start of school in August.

I headed to a common area where I reunited with my parents but didn't see Scott anywhere. We hadn't exchanged phone numbers, and I didn't even know his last name. So I left for home without a goodbye only to resume my part-time job at a small grocery store and summer fling with an older guy, both of which were very temporary. I was eager for the college adventure to begin.

So now it was a couple of months later and I was eating pizza with my new friend in the student center and staring at this guy with whom I'd had such a connection with at the preview weekend. But for the life of me, I couldn't remember his name. Suddenly, our eyes met, and he walked over to my table with those same intense brown eyes and nice legs. He remembered me and my name. (He later confessed that he'd confided to his brother that he'd met a pretty girl named Gina who was very friendly at Preview.)

After he and his new roommate, Brad, joined our table, Scott and I immediately "clicked" again as if no time had passed. We eventually ended up back at my dorm room with Tracy to play cards. I don't remember what card game we played, but I do remember having a huge smile plastered on my face the whole time and how Scott made me feel completely at ease.

While the card playing lasted well into the night, Brad eventually left, and Scott stayed. It was our first day of college, and I barely knew this guy, but I did have a feeling about him. I secretly wished Tracy would leave but I couldn't ask her to do that. So the three of us eventually crashed on my cramped twin bed for an uncomfortable night's sleep.

As we lay side by side with me in the middle, I kept looking back at Scott, letting my eyes tell him that I was completely captivated by him. I pressed my body a little closer to his, but he was a perfect gentleman, and eventually, we all fell asleep.

That night was the beginning of a college romance that lasted all four years. We were inseparable. When I wasn't with him, I was dreaming about him; the feeling was mutual. We had an undeniable chemistry that has continued to this day. Three months after graduation, we were married. Twenty-seven years later, my heart still skips a beat when he walks through the door at the end of the day. And lest we forget, I was the girl who went to college to have *my own* adventure. The last thing on my radar was finding the love of my life that first day on campus. Funny how life happens. We crossed paths several times with Darcy during our college career. On a few occasions we'd pass her in the quad as we strolled hand in hand and exchanged uncomfortable hellos. I always wondered how she felt about the turn of events.

We'd been married just four years when MS reared its ugly head. Twenty-three years later, Scott is still my main support and care partner. He definitely carries more on his broad shoulders than most spouses of healthy partners. In sickness and in health, Scott is steadfastly there for me.

He sees and understands the difficulties I experience doing the simplest tasks. By the time we've prepared a meal together, for example, it's as if I've just completed a marathon. I have to sit down to recharge while he completely takes over serving and cleaning up. He's saddled not only with a full-time job but the laundry, yard work, cleaning that isn't addressed by our cleaning lady, attending sports practices and playing outside with our son, paying the bills, and helping me maneuver through my daily life more and more. He's a hard worker, and fortunately, servitude comes naturally to him. Because of his extra burdens, I encourage him regularly to relax and take time out for himself and do things he enjoys, like cycling, which has become an escape from the daily demands he faces.

I am exceptionally blessed to have always been surrounded by undying love and encouragement — first by the foundation of love and confidence given by my parents and now with the unwavering devotion from my husband and son. It has been nothing less than crucial for my survival with MS. With this kind of support, there is nothing I can't accomplish.

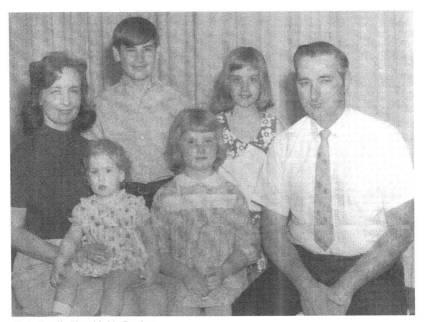

Only Family Pic with My Brother

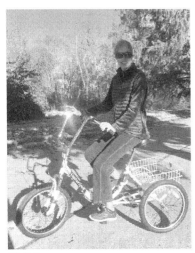

My Trike

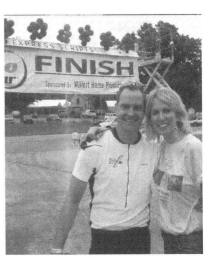

My MS 150 Cyclist Soulmate

CHAPTER TEN

The Greatest Blessing

Difficult roads often lead to beautiful destinations.

~ Zig Ziglar

After marrying and starting our life together, Scott and I were both busy establishing our careers while enjoying carefree fun with little responsibility. We enjoyed fantastic vacations, restaurants, working out together, and eventually building and furnishing our new dream home. We always assumed children would be part of our lives at some point, but early on in our marriage, we weren't interested.

As we witnessed the challenges those around us faced as parents, we often thought child-free, not child-less, might be a worthy option. After all, we'd have less stress, more freedom, and more money without any little people in the picture.

While I was the baby of my family, I wasn't a "baby person." I never felt the need to hold a baby if one was around. New parents would often ask if I wanted to hold their little bambino. While others seem to practically line up for a chance, I was the one who said, "I'm good. Thanks. I can see him from here, and he's adorable!" When babies were happy and cooing, they were cute, but most of the time they seemed messy and undisciplined to me. Scott and I were having a superb time as a couple without the "burden" of children.

We were on a mission to try all of the highly-rated St Louis restaurants in the Zagat guide, and it never failed that we'd encounter a weary-looking couple with baby in tow obviously trying to have a nice meal as they'd done in their pre-parenting days. Instead, they took turns battling with an overtired, whiny child which helped us conclude that parenting looked rather painful.

As the years passed, we checked most everything off our list of things to do except for starting a family. We had a dog, a house, established careers, numerous exotic vacations, so we finally considered the idea of parenthood. While Scott was a kid magnet, they usually steered clear of me. The only saving grace is that both of my older sisters had three children, and I adored being an aunt to all of them. My nieces and nephews melted my heart, so I came to the conclusion that I wasn't completely devoid of the mothering instinct.

We agreed to give it a whirl. Making a baby was supposed to be a simple and enjoyable process. From my perspective, everyone around us seemed to be popping out babies with ease. However, despite discontinuing all birth control measures, nothing happened for us. A few years passed, and while I peed on a few sticks, they never changed colors or made special designs. I read books about "how-to increase your fertility." I charted my temperature to pinpoint ovulation timing. Nothing worked. Though Scott was also attempting obvious fertility-improvement measures, he, at least, wasn't yet a spandex wearing cyclist which could have caused another set of issues.

After all that trying and still no pregnancy, I wondered if my almost forgotten MS diagnosis was to blame. Maybe a hidden sadistic MonSter was inside me playing a cruel joke by attacking my ovaries. The central nervous system and reproductive organs aren't connected, so I knew it didn't make sense but wondered if they'd somehow conspired to sabotage my plans. After this pattern continued for some time, we both underwent fertility testing. Once the results came back, the doc called to say everything was in exemplary working order, and we were diagnosed with "unexplained infertility." That was basically just fancy medical terminology for "we have no idea why you can't make a baby!" All of our parts worked flawlessly on their own, but to our dismay, they weren't interested in collaborating.

While we were confused, we were also relieved and still hopeful that our eggs and swimmers would get together over time, happening when we least expected it. Our doctor suggested taking the next step, but we decided to wait. Even though we felt our parenting clock ticking away, we agreed to remove the pressure and try this thing on our own for a little longer. Armed with proof and with our naturally confident outlooks, there wasn't any reason this shouldn't work!

About that time, a friend of a friend also told me about another friend who had gotten pregnant after seeing a Chinese acupuncturist named Dr.Ginger. She had helped to conceive many babies for other couples like us. One couple was so grateful for her assistance, they named their daughter Ginger after her! Scott and I made an appointment with hopes she would be our pregnancy whisperer. Every other day I went to acupuncture sessions in the city. I changed to an all-natural diet and drank various strange teas and herbal medicine concoctions prescribed by Dr. Ginger. She performed cupping which left horrible bruises making me look like I had been beaten with baseballs. She had me rub my abdomen, feet, and hands every night with a buffalo horn and wear acupressure stickers in my ear to which I applied pressure every four hours. Dr. Ginger often assured me in broken English, "These treat-a-ments will help you get preg-an-ant." As a result, I did whatever she told me to do. After six months of our "last resort" Chinese medicine attempt, we were discouraged. We had spent a few thousand dollars but had no "preg-an-ancy" to show for it. We decided to stop the "treat-a-ments" and take a break. The delay meant that we had more time for vacations and restaurants so we enjoyed both. We got lost in the business of our daily routines and didn't get stuck in the monthly no-pregnancy disappointment. When struggling with infertility, people love to tell you that it will happen once you stop thinking about it so much. Well, it didn't.

After another couple years of negative pregnancy tests, we agreed that maybe we just needed a little medical assistance and decided it was time to pursue artificial insemination. This is when baby making became very unromantic and overly scientific. For six months, we gave it our all. One of the inseminations took place in our doctor's office but mostly the perfect time happened to fall on a weekend when our doc's office was closed. Those months we swapped the starkly cold, drab medical office for a beautifully decorated women's clinic. Surrounded by lit candles and soothing music, we'd lay together for the allotted time following each high-tech injection and hope for the best. As a naturally optimistic person, I fully believed that it was going to work every single time. It never did.

After months of disappointment, we reevaluated. Did we really want to go any further with medical intervention? After all, we were happy as a couple. We were a solid team and maybe this was a sign that we should just forget the idea and move on with our lives. The time, effort, and expense with no "baby-to-be" was wearing on us.

In the meantime, more signs of my MS began surfacing. That's when my bladder became overactive and urgent requiring me to become acutely aware of the location of every clean restroom near any highway in the area. I was stumbling and running into things on a regular basis. I'd been so focused on starting a family that I had forgotten about myself. At Scott's request, I scheduled an appointment with my neurologist. Even though I hadn't seen Dr. G in years, she was one of the most prestigious MS doctors in the area, and Scott was insistent.

At the appointment, I felt immediately connected to my new neurologist. I since learned how important it is to have an open and honest doctor-patient relationship especially with a disease like MS. She took note of my progressed symptoms and ordered a new MRI to be done a few days later. In my almost ten year denial, I had successfully managed to avoid this test but now had to face it again. The harsh and jolting sounds of the first one still echoed in my mind and brought back the memory I'd been avoiding. But since I now knew what to expect, it wasn't as traumatic this time. When this tech rolled me out of the tube, my eyes were dry, and I felt confident and relieved. I had finally conquered that fear!

Around the same time, we opened our minds and explored local adoption agencies. Adoption, like our failed attempt at baby making, seemed to be another drawn out and time-consuming process. We chose our favorite agency and discovered that there was an initial wait of one year just to begin the home study process. Even after waiting the year and crossing the countless hurdles involved, who knew how long the actual baby wait would be. We went ahead and paid our application fee and added our name to the initial waitlist. The agency suggested we consider the foster parent program, but after attending a class and viewing the emotional video (which is most likely used to weed-out those who can't cut it), we skipped that option. Foster parents are very special people, and we instantly realized we weren't up for the emotional challenges involved.

After encouragement from my OB/GYN, we were referred to the next level of fertility specialists. In vitro fertilization (IVF) would be our next medical foray into potential parenthood. We had our first appointment and learned how the process would unfold. At about the same time, we received a call from the adoption agency that it was finally time to start the home study process. We were open to pursuing both options at the same time and would see which one happened first. The mammoth IVF undertaking would begin by attending "shot" class. This class would teach us how to inject my body daily with the necessary lab-created hormonal stimulants to increase the likelihood of a positive result.

We were awake for only a few minutes one morning when my neurologist called. She informed me that the results of

the MRI were back and that I had definite disease progression
with additional plaques on my brain and spinal cord. She
recommended I come into her office immediately to choose
and finally begin one of the injectable medications that were
available to slow further progression. (Ironically, many years
later when I became an MS Advocate speaker, I encouraged
newly diagnosed MS warriors to do the complete opposite
of what I had done upon my diagnosis. Instead of waiting,
they should immediately get started on one of the many MS
therapies now available to potentially slow progression of the
disease.)

After hanging up the phone, Scott and I looked at
each other and immediately knew our plans had just changed
direction again. We skipped the shot class and instead went to
breakfast to weigh the lengthy list of options before us. We drew
them out on a napkin as we waited for pancakes.

a.   If I started on an MS drug therapy, I, of course,
      wouldn't be a candidate for IVF.

b.   If we delayed the suggested drug therapy and pursued
      IVF, we could face months of multiple attempts which
      would mean delaying the treatment I now believed
      necessary.

c.   If we required multiple rounds of IVF, we may not be
      able to afford the expensive MS drug I needed. We
      had no idea whether my insurance would cover any
      of the expensive drugs, and the thought of adjusting

to motherhood while simultaneously managing the possible side effects of an MS drug in my system, scared me to death. Becoming a new mom would be enough of an adjustment!

d.   Even if we underwent several months of this expensive IVF procedure, there was still no guarantee that the goal of a pregnancy would even be achieved. By that time, we could have also blown through any potential adoption funds, leaving us in a worse spot than before.

e.   If we did conceive, who knows how my disease would react to the stress of the inevitable new mom fatigue. We had learned of women with MS who had experienced healthy pregnancies with no exacerbations during the gestation period due to the euphoric effect of pregnancy hormones. After delivery, however, some women's bodies seemed to suffer severe MS relapses and disease progression during those first hectic months of motherhood.

Those were all risks we did not want to take, so at the end of our meal, our decision was made. We would focus all of our energies on the adoption process! After sifting through some initial adoption paperwork, we were immediately thrust into an overwhelming list of requirements. If every potential parent was subjected to these prerequisites, very few would survive the process.

- four parenting and adoption information classes

- multiple individual and couples interviews
- written personal bio and family history autobiographies
- background checks
- home visits
- fingerprinting
- physicals
- at least two recommendation letters for each parent
- album creation complete with lifetime narratives, letters, pictures and bios

When we had our physicals, I hadn't yet begun my MS injections. I purposely visited my GP for the physical exam before that next neuro appointment where I would choose one of the DMDs. That way, I could honestly respond I wasn't currently taking any prescription drugs. This was before the days of electronic record keeping, and since I appeared to be completely healthy with no impaired abilities, the doctor never inquired about my much earlier diagnosis. Call it an error of omission, but he didn't ask, and I didn't tell. Perhaps my years of MS avoidance and disguise were paying off! If the adoption agency would have red-flagged our paperwork noting that the adoptive mother had a chronic progressive illness, who knows what our outcome would have been. A birth mother would, of course, select who received her biological child. An adoptive mom with MS would likely be pushed to the bottom of the pile.

After nine months of time-consuming steps, we were finally ready to enter the waiting game. We were one of several couples on the list and were prepared for a wait that could last up to two years. We were excited and optimistic yet patient. After the marathon we'd just completed, we welcomed the routine of work and normalcy again. Unlike IVF, which you hope will ultimately lead to a baby, we believed that adoption was a sure thing. We were confident that eventually we would be chosen and were all but guaranteed a baby at the end of all this. Since we were done jumping through hoops and navigating red tape, I got Scott's approval to get paint mixed for the baby's room. Prior to that time, he wouldn't agree to decorate a room for a baby that might not exist. He thought it would be depressing to walk by and see a decked out baby-ready room for an indefinite period of time. So, I honored his request (except for when we happened upon a beautiful crib that some toddler parents were purging at a great price). Until I got the green light, that drab white room remained untouched aside from the disassembled crib leaning against the wall and an accumulation of random odds and ends that didn't seem to fit anywhere else in our house.

I'd always loved transforming and decorating a space. Now that I had a crib, I started thinking of paint colors. Scott agreed that a little paint on the walls wouldn't hurt, so I acted quickly before he changed his mind. I visited my local hardware store, chose the perfect samples and had two gallons of paint mixed. Of course, we didn't know if we would end up with a boy or girl, so I planned the colors accordingly: Granny Smith green on bottom, a white chair rail in the middle and a soft sunshine yellow on top. I delivered the paint to the baby's room and wondered if I could enlist Scott and his painting skills to start the project that weekend. We'd only been on the waiting list for a week, so I knew we had plenty of time.

I was working in my home office the next day when my phone rang. It was after lunch, and I'd been on business calls all morning. I was ready to wrap up a few things and get the weekend started early. I gladly picked up the phone thinking it was a friend's number on the ID.

To my surprise, it was our adoption agency caseworker, Sandra. I almost immediately asked her if we had forgotten to sign a required document as there had been countless forms, so it was likely we missed one. She answered my question with a quick no and then asked if I was sitting down. I said I was.

I'll never forget the next sentence as long as I live. It was one of those life-altering moments that becomes eternally emblazoned in your psyche. She said that a birth mom had chosen us to be the parents of her baby boy, and he was due in two weeks!

Time stood still for a few seconds as I absorbed and tried to process her words. My head was swimming! Was this for real? Was I dreaming? Tears of complete joy and shock streamed down my face. We had only been on the waiting list for eight days! I never imagined that it would be that quick. I expected we'd be in a holding pattern for at least a year. She shared a few more details and that she'd be in touch. Yet another life-changing, abruptly ended phone call was on the books!

I dried my eyes, attempted to compose myself, and called Scott at his office. I asked him the same question that Sandra had just asked me. "Are you sitting down?" Then I delivered the news, and we started bawling on the phone together. He stood up screaming and his co-workers rushed to his side asking if everything was okay? After a few hugs and high fives, he headed home so we could cry and scream and hug and jump together!

That weekend was a blur. Filled with complete elation I called everyone I could think of to share our big news. Friends and family were overjoyed for us but were also in shock that it was happening so lightning fast. We were going to be parents in two weeks, and other than some paint and a crib, we had nothing else ready! Scott spent the next 24 hours prepping and painting our soon-to-be son's room without me having to beg. While he brushed and rolled the green and yellow which now could have been blue, I sat in the floor of the now empty room, and we chatted incessantly.

The next day, we ventured out to a monstrous and overwhelming all-things-baby superstore. We had absolutely no idea what any of it was. We didn't have a registry. We didn't know what we needed, and we definitely didn't know where to begin in that maze of a store. We found a friendly clerk who was excited to hear of our impending arrival and willing to help us sort through a very long list of baby necessities. Naturally, we purchased even more than we needed. By Sunday evening, we had finished decorating the room. It was picture perfect and ready for our boy. After that, I joked that I didn't know what everybody else does for nine months.

Over those next two weeks, it was nearly impossible to sleep. I was tired, but my brain wouldn't slow down. As the hours ticked by, I would replay the series of events up until then and envision the gargantuan life change that would unfold in just a matter of days. What kind of mother would I be? Would I adjust to my new life? I also thought about what his birth mom was feeling; was she sure about her decision or would she have second thoughts? After a series of sleepless nights, I began writing letters to my son. It allowed me to therapeutically pour my thoughts on paper. I was writing a letter almost daily and have continued that practice over the years, although much less frequently. They are kept in an album, and we've read many to him as he's gotten older.

One thing we did have planned was a name. If we had a girl, we loved Maya (after Maya Angelou), but if we had a boy, it would be Tristan Maxwell after Brad Pitt's character in *Legends of the Fall* and my dad, Max. When we shared the name with my dad, he responded, "That poor boy!" Maybe he thought the name sounded rather ostentatious or like someone who might get beaten up regularly. Regardless, we realized why many parents don't reveal a name before their soon-to-be babies are born.

We thought we had his name figured out long ago but started considering alternatives. Every suggestion was shot down just as quickly. One day, Scott randomly thought of the name "Reece." I liked it, but Max didn't really work well with it. During a subsequent conversation with my old friend, Carmen, she asked about the baby's name. I relayed the series of events leading to the Reece Max dilemma and almost immediately, she asked about my older brother who had drowned. His name was Max Brand, inspired by the pen name of an author my parents liked. They said the name exuded strength and confidence. The instant the name passed her lips, I knew our son had his name. Reece Brand. Scott agreed, and this time, we kept it a secret from everyone. As the word of our suddenly impending adoption was big family news, we were overwhelmed with love and well wishes. And very quickly, friends, family, and coworkers threw together a beautifully produced baby shower. When we decided to reveal his name at the shower, it was met with an emotional reaction from my mom. Her son would be living on in her grandson, Reece Brand.

In addition to all the shower presents, thoughtful friends delivered gifts and hand-me-downs from children who had outgrown them. We were ready, but he wasn't. Since he waited an extra week to make an appearance, we were able to pull off one last hurrah, a bike ride and winery tour in the country with thoughtful contemplation of what our little guy would be like. I even managed to fit in a previously scheduled business trip to Boston. While there, I was surprised with another celebratory baby shower with friends. This boy certainly had everything he needed, and the anticipation was mounting!

It wasn't until the day before he came into this world that I realized my child had no socks. I freaked out! We had everything imaginable but hadn't considered socks. What kind of parents would we be if we didn't even think of socks? I had other clothing and diapers and wipes and bottles and onesies all laundered and waiting but no socks. Since I was new at this, I didn't realize that newborn babies pretty much live in their little zipper suits with built-in feet, so socks aren't even a necessity for several months. Maybe it was the whirlwind of impending life changes that piqued my emotional sock calamity. I suppose it was just my version of a prenatal meltdown.

As quickly as things happened in those two weeks, it seemed like an eternity waiting for an update once his birth was imminent. Finally at 5:15PM on October 17, 2005, Scott and I received the much anticipated call from the agency! Our son had arrived and was completely healthy with no complications for him or his birth mom. Scott and I were together at the kitchen table trying to absorb every detail of this phone call -- weight, length, exact time of birth, any medical and delivery details, his birth Mom's physical and mental state. Like all of my life-altering phone conversations, it ended quickly and with a promise from our social worker to call the next day with more info.

We were ready to jump in the car and drive the two hours to get him, but there was a state-required waiting period to endure first. He wouldn't be allowed to come home to us for two weeks after leaving the hospital. Additional legal red tape and ad litem guardians were arranged behind the scenes. When we received word that our son was ready to be transferred out of the hospital and we could meet him at his temporary foster home, we hit the road immediately. As we got closer to our destination, our excitement grew. We would be meeting our son for the first time in mere minutes! As we pulled into the neighborhood, we noted the serene and picturesque surroundings. The sun was shining, and the lake behind the sprawling house was glistening. We hadn't imagined such a swank foster home. We barely had a chance to ring the doorbell when the massive door swung open to reveal several smiling faces, one of which was handing me a beautiful baby boy wrapped in a light green blanket. I was holding my son! He was really mine! Scott and I were euphoric as we took turns holding him. We even unwrapped him to count and check out his little fingers and toes.

The birth mom's social worker was there and told us how the process had quickly unfolded. When she came to the adoption agency just a few weeks before her delivery, she was very clear about her decision. If we had delayed or taken one extra week to finalize our paperwork, this serendipitous match would not have happened. Our file hadn't even been completely finalized when our caseworker, Sandra, saw the birth mom's preferences come through the agency's computer system and made sure our album was presented.

The birth mom had somehow kept the pregnancy a secret from everyone around her, getting herself to the hospital and through the ensuing birthing process alone. We already admired her, and the feeling of gratitude soared as we learned more about her.

We cried and laughed and took pictures, but eventually, it was time to leave. What a bizarre feeling it was to meet our son and then head home empty handed. Fantasies of running to the car with him in our arms crossed our minds, but we knew a kidnapping charge would only compromise our ultimate goal. They already knew everything about us, down to our address and blood types, so the chances of being incognito were unlikely. Our only solace was feeling exceedingly comfortable with his foster family. They were remarkable people who loved babies and had two toddlers of their own. They knew what they were doing and seemed to enjoy every minute. They told us about picking him up from the hospital and what a sweet baby he had been so far. They wanted to be of help during this time of transition and said we could come back to visit anytime. They even offered us use of their entire lower level, which was like a small house, to hang out in as a family until we could bring him home in two weeks. We went as often as possible. They gave us space to be alone, even leaving the house as they continued with the busy requirements of their active family. During our visits, we learned valuable tips from their years of baby experience. They taught us how to bathe him and shared a play by play account of his life between our visits.

We got to meet Reece's birth mom a couple weeks later. She was in college at the time, and this was definitely not part of her future plan. She was friendly and smart, and at a different time and under different circumstances, she and I might have become close friends. We spoke easily, and she even shared the reasons she chose us. Just one other couple included a birth-Mom letter but only ours showed any interest and concern for her difficult situation. She also appreciated that our album was well composed and not riddled with grammatical errors like others. She was a grammar Nazi like me, and I was ecstatic that my writing skills had helped secure her decision! The profile pic with our cute little Pekingese sealed the deal. We learned bits and pieces about her family and life at college. She said she was initially in disbelief about the pregnancy and kept it a secret from those closest to her which reminded me of my own denial and attempted cover up of MS. Even though she didn't seek medical care until she was nearly in the third trimester, she had taken excellent care of herself during the pregnancy. She had eaten well, continued to jog and avoided alcohol. She wanted to make sure this baby was healthy.

Before meeting her, we racked our brains to settle on a present that would adequately express our gratitude for the monumental gift she was giving us. Nothing seemed worthy. What would a 19 year-old girl treasure? My friend, Christina, had two teenage daughters and knew that Tiffany-blue packaging was guaranteed to get a positive reaction. We settled on a Tiffany bracelet, and she was ecstatic. She seemed as overjoyed to receive the bracelet as we were to be handed her biological son. We will always honor this brave young woman who gave us the most precious gift one human can grant another. I am eternally grateful she was allowed to make that very personal decision herself and wasn't forced into it, choosing to carry our son to full term. We are forever thankful and indebted to her.

A few years ago in a Target parking lot, my son asked me this question out of the blue. "So, if I didn't come out of your belly, whose belly did I come out of?" I was pulling out of my parking space when he threw this curveball of a question at me. I thought for a moment before answering simply and honestly, "She was a wonderful young woman who chose me and dad to be your parents." He let that sink in and then responded, "Wow, she must have been really smart because she made a great choice!" That was it. Then he moved on to wondering about lunch plans. His birth mom had expressed her hope for him to be a great communicator. Mission accomplished.

Reece is quite comfortable with being adopted. In a

recent conversation he asked, "So if Grandpa has Alzheimer's and you have MS, and I'm adopted, does that mean that I DON'T have your genes?" I responded, "That's true. You don't." With a look of pure exhilaration complete with a huge grin and powerful fist pump, he exclaimed, "YES!"

In the 13 years since our son was born, he not only continues to amaze, delight, and inspire us, but he takes great joy in making me laugh. He doesn't just go for those under my breath chuckles. No, his goal is to render me gasping and hyperventilating, bent over and crying. Not only is he savagely witty, wise, sarcastic, and fun, but he's exceedingly talented, confident, and fearless as he attempts new endeavors. Scott is all about sports, and I was always wordy and musical, so it's fitting that he excels at all of those things. He's played soccer and now gravitates more to baseball and basketball. As for musical instruments, he began with and continues piano in addition to trumpet, guitar, a French horn stint, and most recently, drums. On top of all that, he's also an academic achiever and exceptionally cute. Can you tell I'm a proud momma?

Most of all, the kindness and empathy he's developed, undoubtedly due in part to having a mother with special needs, has given him an extraordinarily big heart. He's the one who has seen me fall more than anyone else. He always rushes to my side to ask if I'm okay and helps me get back on my feet. As he's gotten older, he's become a great help to me and his father. Now when we're out and about, he often waits for me, bending his arm at a 90-degree angle just like his dad so I can stabilize myself. He's learning great determination by watching me persevere and push forward with a joyful attitude in spite of my stumbles. He is also keenly aware of the times when I get frustrated with my lack of ability to do what I wish I could do. During those rare moments, he's great at encouraging and comforting -- all signs of a sensitive and compassionate soul. My love for him is full and never ending, and he hears that daily. The last words he hears each day before catching the school bus are inspired by *The Help*: You are smart, you are kind, and you are very important. While our path to parenthood may have involved adjusting, recalculating, and maneuvering through non-conventional hurdles, the end result couldn't have been any sweeter.

Here is part of a letter I penned to him two weeks before he arrived.

Saturday, 10-01-2005

Hello Again Reece,

Your Grandma and Grandpa Whitlock came over today to visit and see your room. They were impressed with how beautiful it is. We shopped for more baby things and they purchased a changing table for your room.

I have tons of nervous energy and have noticed myself

talking faster and buzzing around in a state of constant motion.
I haven't slept past 5 am since I heard the news so I guess I'm
getting ready for all the sleepless nights with you.

We have so many hopes and dreams for you! We promise
to cheer when you achieve even the smallest accomplishments
and hold your hand when you stumble and fall. We plan to model
for you how to communicate positively and effectively -- both
verbally and written -- to guarantee you have strong relationships
throughout your life. We hope to instill in you a respect for
authority -- especially for your parents, grandparents, and
teachers. We want to show you how to appreciate diversity as
you come into contact with others of different races, backgrounds,
religions or classes. We want to help you dream and instill in you
the knowledge that if you dream it and are willing to work hard,
*then you can achieve it. We don't want you to become what _we_*
desire but instead we want you to discover your own passions.
Whatever it is that you decide to pursue, we will encourage you
to work hard and do your very best at it. And, most importantly,
we hope you watch how your parents interact and treat each
other with love, patience and respect so that you will have a
better chance at finding and maintaining the same kind of loving
relationship that we have.

We know that someday, you may have questions about
your birth parents -- that's only natural. While we have very
limited information about them, we do know that your Birth Mom
was courageous in making her adoption plan for you. She put
her concerns for your future above anything else. She knew that

she was unable to give you the best that life has to offer and was willing to make the biggest sacrifice a woman can make...We thank her daily for the insight, love and concern she had for you and will always be indebted to her for that.

Now the clock is ticking as we wait for your birth and we are caught up in buying baby gear and all the necessary accoutrements. But in the back of our minds we wonder, like all new parents must, how we are going to figure this all out. We don't know how to heat up bottles and fasten car seats and bathe a newborn and choose the right formula and on and on. But we DO know how to LOVE you and that is the one sure thing that we come back to in those moments of panic. We hope that someday when you read this letter, you will understand what we went through to bring you into our lives and just how special and important that makes you. All good things are worth waiting for and we love you Reece Brand Fletcher more than you will ever know!

> *With all our love,*
> *Mom and Dad*

Not Flesh of My Flesh, nor bone of my bone but still miraculously my own. Never forget for a single minute, you didn't grow under my heart but in it. ~ Fleur Conkling Heyliger

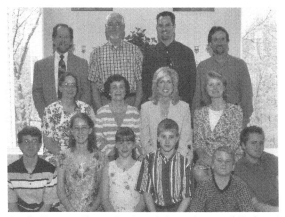
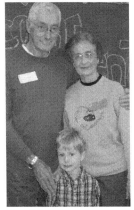

Family (Parents, Sisters, Brothers-in-law, Nieces and Nephews)   *Proud Grandparents*

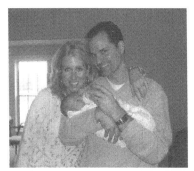
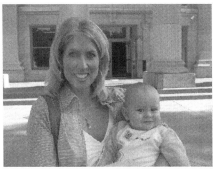

Meeting Reece   *Adoption Finalized*

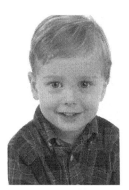
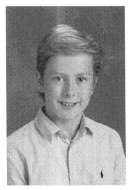

Reece, 2 years old   *Reece, 12 years old*

CHAPTER ELEVEN

Time to Rise

Kites rise highest against the wind - not with it.
~ Winston Churchill

My central nervous system has gone haywire and completely changed my life. Fluctuating this way and that between frustration, joy, anger, laughter, and sadness, I've been forced to mourn the loss of my former active self. Oh, what I wouldn't give to once again take long walks with my husband, strolling hand in hand together through our neighborhood or through a park, enjoying the fresh air as we solved the world's problems. Such a seemingly simple thing is but a treasured memory. I fondly remember exploring different neighborhoods and catching cable cars on the hilly streets of San Francisco and the joy of meandering down a sandy beach without worrying about my stability on the uneven sand or my bladder suddenly crying out for relief. Just wearing a pair of sexy and stylish stilettos would be a thrill. All of those things seem like part of a stranger's foggy memory now. What perhaps breaks my heart more than anything these days is my inability to run, hike, play catch, and shoot baskets with my highly active 13-year-old son.

This disease has robbed me of much, but being grateful for the abilities I do have rather than resentful about what I don't, is a necessity when dealing with adversity. If I chose to constantly dwell on what I've lost, I would probably never get out of bed. In addition to practicing conscious gratitude, I've become an expert at coping with a disease that's like climbing up a steep, never-ending, earth-sized mountain covered in twisted vines covering hidden, random potholes with a 500 pound weight on my back as my legs wobble and crash to the ground periodically from fatigue. As a result of this gargantuan daily effort, my mind must maintain the strength and positive perspective which my disease attempts to stifle. MS may have stolen my abilities, but it won't take away my joyful outlook.

In computer science, the principle of "garbage in, garbage out" means that inputting flawed data will generate a low quality output. If you compile a database of all the addresses in your neighborhood but enter the incorrect house numbers, your address book is worthless. I've found the same theory holds true for my perspective. I find more strength, gratitude and belief in myself and others when I read uplifting books and messages and listen to music that makes me happy or podcasts and TV shows that inspire me or make me laugh. Of course, choosing to surround myself with like-minded folks and avoiding those who bring me down are all things that improve my mindset. It all starts in my head. Where my mind goes is where my energy flows. If all that I can see is what I lack, then I will get stuck in that dark place. Like those yellow cars, I find what I look for. Happiness and joy are not dependant on perfect circumstances but instead are the results of making the choice regardless of the cards you've been dealt.

I remember whining a few times to my mom through the years. She listened but usually followed with her own brand of insight, "Well, it could be worse." Then she would go into a story explaining how so-and-so had it far worse than me. Though I sometimes just wanted a little motherly sympathy, her perspective has influenced me greatly. Ironically, when I've complained about my uncooperative legs, my own son has responded just like his Grandma Marion. "Mom, at least you have legs. Some kids aren't even born with legs, and they figure it out."

Like my wise mom and son mused, I'm not the only one struggling, and no matter what, it *could* be worse. Of course, I miss my pre-MS life, but if we only look backwards, we miss out on the happiness surrounding us right now. When I speak to audiences of people who are dealing with adversity, I end every talk with this Eleanor Roosevelt quote: "Yesterday is history. Tomorrow is a mystery. Today is a gift."

None of us are promised any more than this moment. No one knows the future. MS is unpredictable, but so is everything else in this life. I will be in the exact same spot whether I choose to be grateful for what I have, or remorseful about what I don't. I choose my outlook, and life is much more enjoyable when I choose gratitude, savoring all that I have, rather than mourning what's gone.

So, to keep me motivated and looking forward instead of looking back, these three things have become my driving force:

- Focus on taking control of what I CAN control while replacing worry with HUMOR.
- Realize that everyone is dealing with challenges. MS just happens to be mine. I lead my life. I don't let my challenge / my disease lead me
- Be grateful for the many blessings in my life and celebrate them daily while remembering the simple law of attraction -- what I focus on expands.

I've found the saying "perception is reality" to be very true. What I focus on really does increase. When I allowed myself to feel the abundance of what I had, finding even more of it seemed to happen organically and with ease.

According to Overcomingms.org, depression is even

more common for people with MS than for people with other chronic illnesses, with approximately half of all people with MS suffering from depression at some point during their lifetime. Even more eye opening is that for people with MS, depression is the single most important factor affecting quality of life – even more so than disability or fatigue. Chronic conditions, troubled relationships, or floundering careers all worsen when depression is in the picture. Just like using a cane or walker, there shouldn't be shame in seeking needed professional help or antidepressants to get through it. All necessary tools for many. For me, my father's optimistic outlook laid the foundation for developing a gratitude and law-of-attraction mindset which was a powerful antidote to depression. I also credit my ambitious career pursuits with establishing a forward-thinking viewpoint. Even though frustrations grew as my abilities became impaired, I had a driving force pushing me forward each day. There was simply no time to dwell on my worsening symptoms. My distraction of busyness help me avoid anxious despair. Feeling productive, successful, and helpful to others benefitted my situation. As progressing symptoms finally forced me out of that career, I believed that even though one part of my life was ending, something else would appear. As one door closed, I knew that another would present itself but had no idea what it might be. When I was deep into my business, I became a big fan of sticky notes. Over the years, I began using them to post positive reminders and messages on my computer, my steering wheel, the bathroom mirror -- anywhere I'd see regularly.

When pain became the center of my existence and was so intense it regularly brought tears to my eyes, I needed a more organized and measured way to keep a healthy perspective. Toiling in daily misery made for a dismal existence. I needed a reboot and moved from sticky notes to "Gratitude Journaling." I found a notebook, kept it handy on the nightstand for easy access, and made my first entry:

1. I woke up today
2. My pain was a little less than yesterday
3. Watching a silly movie with Scott while Reece napped was a great distraction

When this journaling process was new, I doubted whether I would have much to record. When you're in a funk, gratitude does not come easily. I started anyway, simply aiming to write in the notebook every day. After a month, I formed a habit. When I reviewed my entries, I was amazed at how much easier it had become to find more to be thankful for in each day. I realized I am what I think about, and when I spent time regularly reflecting on the good, then more of it seemed to find its way to me. Eventually, gratitude, became a natural daily habit like brushing my teeth.

But, of course, dental hygiene didn't begin as a natural habit either. My son is now 13 and teeth brushing is finally ingrained. Until recently, I would ask him if he had remembered and most days he would say, "Oh yeah, I forgot." Becoming gratitude-centered is the same. It flexes a muscle that becomes stronger and habitual the more it's used. Just like using prayer and meditation as moments of pause, I used the gratitude journal to form a muscle-building habit. Like the letters I wrote while waiting for Reece, the journaling process quickly became cathartic. Putting thoughts on paper also triggered a memory of my love of writing...

For most of my adult life, I haven't had a hobby. I never painted, took photos, scrapbooked, climbed mountains, or crocheted. Instead, I focused on work, my health, raising a family, keeping a home in order, and maintaining a happy marriage. Who had time for other interests? If someone asked what I did in my spare time, I would share the rote answer that I enjoyed spending time with family and friends.

When my parents moved into an assisted living center and my sisters and I removed the final remnants of childhood from the family home, I found decades-old stories I'd written in the boxes of school papers and memories which my sentimental mother had lovingly preserved. As I read them, my elementary school dream of becoming a children's book author came rushing back. I had to admit, the stories seemed well written for a child that age. I enjoyed showing them to my son as he strained to imagine his mom actually being a kid once upon a time. After a weekend walking down memory lane, I eventually grew tired of the mess in the dining room and returned the stories to their plastic tote to be hidden away indefinitely in the basement like so many things from our past that don't quite fit into our current life.

Still, I was reminded of my youthful love of writing. Unlike most of my classmates, I always looked forward to writing essays. I was the nerd who took great pleasure in diagramming sentences (a skill today's youth will never learn). My elementary school teacher, Mrs. Gregory, could attest to my adoration of the English language.

In college I took a Women in Literature class that I loved. When my then boyfriend, now husband, needed a senior year English credit, I encouraged him to take that same class since I thought he'd find it as engaging as I had. I was wrong. It wasn't his cup of tea. When the final paper was due and he was completely stumped, I offered to lend a hand. Not my proudest moment, but I ran with it and took great joy in writing about Jane Austen's, *The Awakening*.

When the professor distributed copies of "his" paper to the entire class the following week, Scott was dumbfounded. The teacher was using "his" essay as an example of how to write an impactful paper. In fact, he asked Scott if he could submit the essay for publication to a Chicago-based literary magazine. When Scott told me, I was thrilled! I was going to be published! But then I quickly realized that none of it was possible. Our unethical move had proven again that dishonesty sucks. My disappointment and sadness were real as Scott convincingly explained to his professor that he only wrote the paper for personal enjoyment and wasn't interested in having it published.

Even when my mother passed away last year, I realized how therapeutic it was to put words on paper. Though I was ugly-crying while I wrote her eulogy, the process brought me a bit of peace during a sad time.

Rewind to several years earlier when I barely started this book. After only a few pages, I stopped. I was too busy to write. I had daily lists of things to do with goals to reach, and writing didn't fit into my schedule. Besides, my tremoring hands and failed grip not only made writing with a pen and paper nearly impossible, but also made typing a challenge. Also, being hunched over the computer for long periods of time was uncomfortable and intensified my MS Hug pain. Periodically my son would ask if I was still writing that "Stumble" book, but my answer was always the same. "Not yet Bud. I will someday." Once again I was letting go of my dream as I doubted I could ever finish a book. Then one day he suggested trying voice-activated typing. I was ecstatic! This simple method made "writing" physically possible again. Once I started speaking the words, my book came to life. Like many times before, it was clear that I wouldn't have to give up my goal just because the obvious path was blocked.

Around that same time, my sister, Becca, and her

husband were down for a rare weekend visit. While in the middle of making a special meal for them, my feet got tangled and I stumbled into the very hard granite corner of our kitchen counter. No one saw the mishap, and my elevated threshold for pain enabled me to plow ahead and finish preparing the meal without any mention. It wasn't until Monday morning that Scott learned of my collision with the granite. When he gave me a hug as he left for work, I recoiled in severe pain. He insisted we go immediately to our friendly urgent care. Of course, wouldn't you know, the x-ray glaringly showed a broken rib and bruised lung.

I was in pain and received doctors' orders to rest and recoup for six weeks. After a couple of days playing with my phone and watching TV, I stationed myself in a recliner and "wrote" feverishly, talking this entire book into a Google doc like my smart son suggested. I remembered how much I enjoyed the writing process, and I couldn't stop. Maybe I could finish a book! While I never thought of writing as a hobby, I do know it's something I enjoy and do fairly well. The passion that writing has renewed in me has been overwhelming. I find myself lying awake at night thinking about the next chapter or my next book. While I don't relish sleep loss, it's incredibly powerful to uncover something that gets your mind firing with excitement and creativity. Finding or rediscovering your "thing" can provide a renewed focus and may even provide a much-needed refuge. With MS challenges, it's easy to get caught up in that downward spiral. You can easily forget who you were or could be in the midst of all the insanity of flare ups, increasing disability, treatment options, and insurance companies while still juggling the regular demands of work and family.

When I re-read the first draft of my original book, I realized I'd written those words before many parts of my life had transformed. Transformation is one of my favorite words since it can mean that new beginnings are created. MS might be the reason I had to transform, but if so, I'm grateful to this disease for pointing me in a new direction that's brought revitalized energy and passion to my life as an author and inspirational speaker. As we are all just here for a short time, I'm hopeful about continuing to thrive in a new direction. Writing has opened up a whole new world of possibilities for me, and I hope it might also inspire others to look at making adjustments or considering other options when their current situation is no longer viable.

MS has not made me weak. In fact, I now realize that the opposite is true. It's revealed to me strength I never imagined I had. Despite many stumbles, I've been forced to recalculate, adjust, and move on while navigating new pathways to achieve my goals. I've taken 100% responsibility for my health and my happiness with no grudges or regrets. I can proudly attest to the astounding benefits of surrounding myself with supportive people and tools while embracing a gratitude-centered mindset.

As I continue through this magical life at peace with a disease I didn't choose, I look at the world through my Dad's eyes. The world is indeed full of mostly good and, like him, I choose to see it each day. When I search my less-than-ideal conditions for joy, kindness, wonder, and possibilities, I find them everywhere. If my lens becomes temporarily clouded by blame, fear, or ego, those lonely burdens are all I see. It's easier now to self-correct when my mind goes to a gloomy place. I don't get stuck there. I choose joy, gratitude, and abundance. I am completely imperfect and find solace and compassion in knowing the same holds true for everyone around me and across this planet. Forever and always we humans have been struggling, floundering, learning, loving, searching, and doing our best. We are not toiling alone! It's refreshing to find the commonalities and even humor in all of our imperfections. As I continue to fight my battle, I can proudly look back and say that I had to STUMBLE in order to RISE. I expect, however, that I will continue to learn from the best teacher -- my future stumbles. As long as my breath goes in and out, I'll be traveling the journey each day with an open mind and a joyful heart.

Stumbling is inevitable. Rising, however, is optional. ~ Gina Whitlock Fletcher

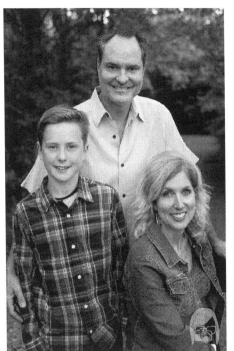

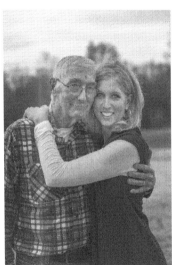

My Greatest Influence

Our Family 2018

Conclusion

This story of my life with MS is just that -- my own story. I've heard this disease described accurately as a multidimensional snowflake. With more than 2.3 million people affected by MS worldwide, I'm convinced there are that many variations of this disease. My experience is completely my own and very different than others with MS. In turn, what works for me may not work for someone else. The good news for any of us dealing with this unpredictable disease at this time in history is that much research and resources abound.

Not so many years ago, the "hot bath" test was used to diagnose multiple sclerosis. A person suspected of having the condition was immersed in a hot tub of water, and the appearance or worsening of neurologic symptoms was taken as evidence the person had MS.[8]

An MS diagnosis meant your life would never be the

---

8   https://www.nationalmssociety.org/Living-Well-With-MS/Diet-
         Exercise-Healthy-Behaviors/Heat-Temperature-Sensitivity

same. Patients were told to take it easy and essentially give in to their situation. They shouldn't expect much of a future as their new life would now revolve around rest and declining health.

When I was diagnosed in 1995, the understanding of MS was still limited. I'm certain that if I were diagnosed now, my disease experience would have been radically different. These days, doctors, and patients make a plan together to treat the disease as aggressively and quickly as possible.

Research is making significant strides to improve, prevent, and modify the likelihood of being diagnosed with MS and if so, to impact disease progression. [9] Fortunately, progress leads to more progress. Much credit goes to the National Multiple Sclerosis Society for becoming the largest private funder of MS research in the world. Teams are studying causation and progression due to genetic factors, virus exposure, effects of smoking and vitamin D levels, obesity in adolescence, gut microbiomes, and biomarkers of the protein neurofilament light chain (NFL) levels, just to name a few. Yes, science is also finally exploring how MS, diet and exercise are interrelated!

No longer are steroids the main line of defense as in the old days. Organizations like Can Do MS are encouraging physical movement and healthy modifications to promote a better outcome for both patients and caregivers once diagnosis has happened.

Local support and exercise groups, online tools, Facebook groups, Podcasts, YouTube channels, and hopefully

9   https://multiplesclerosisnewstoday.com/

friends and family are all important resources that are continually expanding and evolving. This disease is no longer a lonely one.

In the age of technology and personal handheld devices, those things can either serve to divide and isolate or connect and bring together. Like the theme of my book, it's up to each of us to build the supportive networks we need. By taking 100% responsibility for our awareness and outlook we find helpful resources are there. It's up to us to seek them out.

Until MS is eradicated, I will do my part to maintain current abilities while putting up a fight against worsening of this condition. And most of all, I'm committed to spreading awareness and light for others dealing with their own stumbles.

ACKNOWLEDGMENTS

Nothing of significance was ever achieved by an individual acting alone. Look below the surface and you will find that all seemingly solo acts are really team efforts. ~ John Maxwell

Becoming an author has forever been on my radar but felt out of reach as I juggled life's demands. It's funny how the things that we wholeheartedly *want* to do get brushed aside by the things we *have* to do. When a lifelong desire is finally attained, the reward is especially satisfying. Most goals worth reaching don't happen though without great effort, support, and sacrifice. Yes, I'm the writer, but there is a whole tribe of stand-up people I love and appreciate behind the curtain. They've helped me steer through the moving parts of taking this book that was hidden in my phone to a bound and beautiful dream come true.

Much appreciation goes out to my two big sisters, Becca and Laura, for rallying around me -- offering their honest input, intellect and laughs. Our three-way conversations bring me joy and comfort especially when looking for sympathy and giggles following my latest stumble.

My brother-in-law Jerry, deserves not only mucho thanks but many bags of chips for his contribution to making me a better writer throughout every stage of this constantly morphing project. Farming and writing don't typically go hand-in-hand, but he's an exception. Kudos to my other brother-in-law, Kevin, for his techie skills that saved me hours of frustration. Yes, my sisters both married well. And thanks also to my nieces (by blood and marriage), Lauren and Sarah, who graciously lent me their talents of photography and initial cover design and brainstorming. Much gratitude to my fellow-writer and kind-hearted high school friend, Kathy, for her time, insight, and editing skills. I'm honored that this project has reconnected us in such a personal way. Also, her introduction to cover design diva, Shelby, was but fate. Meeting Stephen at the end of the book journey to help me tie all of the pieces together was the finishing touch. I began this book with complete faith that it would somehow all fall into place like a beautiful symphony. I had no idea how this would happen. Thanks to you all, it did, and I am forever indebted.

I'm saddened that my book-loving parents aren't able to witness how I've reinvented myself. In addition, they would be proud of the family effort that has contributed to this project. I'll forever hold a deep gratitude for the inspiration, confidence, and constant love they provided.

High fives and fist pumps all around for my wise, visionary son, Reece. He inspires me daily. Because of his encouragement, this book came to life.

I owe my other half, Scott, for tolerating endless hours absorbed by my new love -- writing. I now have a match for his biking and football obsessions. The gratitude I have for him, however, goes much deeper. As my "person" and caregiver he carries a hefty load with my lengthy list of requirements and needed assistance that most men couldn't bear. I was high maintenance before MS, but now it's climbed to a whole new level. He jumps in with a smile where I fall short. At the end of each day he's the one I want to chill out with and love.

It has truly taken a village, and that makes the end result even sweeter.

Pay It Forward

Gina looks forward to inspiring others through her writing and speaking. She's been described by audiences as an "Inspirational and Relatable Obstacle Overcomer." To share your book feedback, insights, or to inquire about arranging for Gina to write or speak to your group, please send your email to GinaWFAuthor@gmail.com. You can support this independent author by leaving a review on Amazon, following Gina at StumbletoRise.com, and recommending this book to your friends. The best gift you can give is suggesting *Stumble to Rise* to someone who's struggling. As all of us are navigating through some kind of muck, let's support one another as we learn and rise together.

Made in the USA
Columbia, SC
22 April 2019